THE COMPLETE 2024 LOW RESIDUE DIET COOKBOOK

A Comprehensive Beginners Guide for Managing Digestive Disorder and Delicious Anti-Inflammatory Recipes for Healthy Gut

LUCKY WILSON

Copyright © 2024 by Lucky Wilson

All rights reserved. No part of this publication may be reproduced, distributed, or transmitted in any form or by any means, including photocopying, recording, or other electronic or mechanical methods, without the prior written permission of the publisher, except in the case of brief quotation embodied in critical reviews and certain other noncommercial uses permitted by copyright law.

Table of Contents

INTRODUCTION 9

    Understanding the Low Residue Diet 9

    Benefits of a Low Residue Diet 11

    Essential Tips for Following a Low Residue Diet 14

Foods to Avoid and Foods to Eat on a Low Residue Diet. 17

    Foods to Avoid 17

    Foods to Eat 19

Breakfast Delights for Low Residue Diet 21

Lunch Favorites for a Low Residue Diet 23

Dinner Ideas for a Low Residue Diet 26

Snack Options for a Low Residue Diet 28

Side Dishes and Add-Ons for a Low Residue Diet 31

Desserts and Treats for a Low Residue Diet 33

Drinks and Beverages for a Low Residue Diet 35

Meal Plans and Shopping Lists for a Low Residue Diet ... 38

Low residue diet Recipes 42

    Chicken Breast in White Sauce (Low Fat) 42

Low fodmap chili con carne 45

Low Carb Greek Yoghurt Chicken 47

Low Carb Egg Drop Soup 48

The Best Keto Cheese Sauce 50

Easy vegan chickpea curry 51

Low Calorie Chicken and Veggies Stir Fry 53

GLUTEN-FREE COCONUT CHICKEN CURRY RECIPE (LOW FODMAP + DAIRY FREE) 55

Lemon Chicken Rice Soup 59

Chicken Breast in White Sauce (Low Fat) 60

Roasted Squash and Parmigiano Reggiano Stuffed Pasta 63

Low-Residue Turmeric Fish With Baked Sweet Potato and Avocado 66

Zucchini Noodles With Ginger-Peanut Sauce 68

RAW APPLE CARROT CAKE 70

RICE CONGEE 71

Pasta Bake 72

Spinach & Mushroom Quiche 74

TURMERIC CHICKEN AND SWEET POTATO THAI CURRY 75

Lean Meat and Chicken Stew with Chunky Vegetables (Low-Residue Diet) 77

Healthy Low Fat Fried Rice 79

Stir-Fry Velveted Chicken and Vegetables 80

Fruity sponge cake 83

Low Residue Low Fiber Chicken Vegetable Pasta Soup 84

Greek Yogurt Fettuccini Alfredo 85

Low-Residue Turmeric Fish With Baked Sweet Potato and Avocado 87

Tummy Friendly Creamy Pumpkin Soup 88

Low FODMAP Potato Salad 90

Spanish-Style Shrimp Paella 93

CLEAR SOUP RECIPE (CLEAR VEGETABLE SOUP) 95

Low FODMAP Pasta Sauce 98

Low Residue Low Fiber Chicken Vegetable Pasta Soup 100

Low Residue Low Fiber Beet Carrot Soup 101

Greek Yogurt Fettuccini Alfredo 102

Super Simple Gnocchi and Avocado Bake (Low-Residue) 105

Healthy Fried Rice Recipe 106

Low FODMAP Cottage Pie 108

Roasted asparagus 111

Low fodmap pasta sauce 112

Garlic and onion-free taco seasoning 113

Low Residue Smoothie Recipes 115

Triple Berry Oat Smoothie 115

Banana-Oat Smoothie 116

Dairy-Free Strawberry-Banana Smoothie 117

Easy 5 Minute Banana Smoothie 118

Banana Coconut Smoothie 119

Banana Berry Smoothie 119

Strawberry High-Protein Fruit Smoothie 120

Banana Bread Smoothie 121

Healthy Chocolate Banana Smoothie 122

Keto Smoothie Recipe With Avocado, Chia Seeds & Cacao 123

GREEN PROTEIN POWER BREAKFAST SMOOTHIE 124

Oats Smoothie for Weight Loss 126

GUT FRIENDLY SMOOTHIE 128

Strawberry and Banana Fruit Smoothie 129

The Best High Fiber Smoothie (Easy + Healthy) 130

Banana, oat and blueberry breakfast smoothie 131

Fruit & Yogurt Smoothie 132

Peanut Butter and Jelly Smoothie 133

Pumpkin and Turmeric Smoothie 134

Low Sugar Simple Green Smoothie 134

Healthy Green Smoothie 137

Low Sugar Simple Green Smoothie 139

Detox Smoothie 141

EASY DETOX SMOOTHIE 143

30 Days Meal Plan for Low Residue 145

CONCLUSION...156

INTRODUCTION

Understanding the Low Residue Diet

A low residue diet is designed to reduce the amount of undigested food that passes through the intestines, thereby minimizing stool production and alleviating symptoms in individuals with digestive disorders. This diet is particularly beneficial for people with conditions such as Crohn's disease, ulcerative colitis, diverticulitis, or those recovering from bowel surgery. By limiting fiber intake, the diet aims to ease the digestive process and reduce bowel movements.

The primary focus of a low residue diet is to restrict foods that are high in fiber, including whole grains, nuts, seeds, raw fruits, and vegetables. Instead, the diet emphasizes easily digestible foods such as white bread, rice, pasta, and well-cooked vegetables. Proteins like tender meat, fish, and eggs are also encouraged, as they are low in fiber and easier on the digestive system. Dairy products can be consumed in moderation, provided they do not exacerbate symptoms.

While following a low residue diet, it is essential to maintain balanced nutrition. This can be challenging due to the exclusion of many nutrient-rich foods. Therefore, it's important to plan meals carefully to ensure adequate intake of essential vitamins and minerals. Supplements may be necessary to meet nutritional needs, particularly for vitamins A, C, and folate, which are commonly found in high-fiber foods.

Adhering to a low residue diet can significantly improve quality of life for those with certain gastrointestinal conditions. By reducing the volume and frequency of stools, this diet helps minimize discomfort and allows the intestines to heal. However, it is generally intended for short-term use during flare-ups or recovery periods. Long-term adherence without medical supervision can lead to nutritional deficiencies and other health issues.

A low residue diet is a therapeutic approach that eases the burden on the digestive system by limiting fiber intake. It provides relief for individuals with specific gastrointestinal conditions, but careful planning and medical guidance are crucial to ensure nutritional adequacy and avoid potential deficiencies.

Benefits of a Low Residue Diet

The low residue diet offers several benefits, particularly for individuals suffering from digestive disorders. By reducing the intake of high-fiber foods, this diet can significantly alleviate symptoms and improve overall digestive health. Here are some key benefits:

1. Reduces Bowel Movements and Eases Diarrhea: One of the primary benefits of a low residue diet is the reduction in stool volume and frequency. This can be particularly helpful for individuals with conditions like Crohn's disease or ulcerative colitis, where frequent and urgent bowel movements are common. By consuming low-fiber foods,

the digestive system processes less bulk, leading to fewer and more manageable bowel movements. This can also help in easing diarrhea, providing much-needed relief.

2. Minimizes Abdominal Pain and Cramping: High-fiber foods can cause increased gas production and bloating, which often leads to abdominal pain and cramping. A low residue diet, by focusing on easily digestible foods, helps to minimize these symptoms. This is particularly beneficial for individuals with irritable bowel syndrome (IBS) or diverticulitis, where reducing discomfort is a key aspect of managing the condition.

3. Facilitates Intestinal Healing: For those recovering from bowel surgery or experiencing flare-ups of inflammatory bowel diseases, a low residue diet can promote intestinal healing. By limiting fiber, the diet reduces mechanical irritation and allows the inflamed or damaged intestines to heal more effectively. This can accelerate recovery and reduce the risk of complications.

4. Improves Nutrient Absorption: Digestive disorders can often impair the body's ability to absorb nutrients. A low residue diet, by minimizing the presence of undigested food in the intestines, can enhance nutrient absorption. This is

crucial for maintaining overall health and preventing deficiencies that could exacerbate the underlying condition.

5. Reduces Risk of Bowel Obstruction: In individuals with strictures or narrowings in the intestines, a low residue diet can help prevent bowel obstructions. High-fiber foods can form large, bulky stools that may struggle to pass through these narrowed areas. By consuming low-fiber, easy-to-digest foods, the risk of blockages is significantly reduced, preventing painful and potentially serious complications.

6. Provides Relief During Flare-Ups: For chronic conditions like Crohn's disease or ulcerative colitis, flare-ups can be particularly challenging. A low residue diet offers a practical dietary strategy to manage these periods, providing relief from symptoms and reducing the severity of flare-ups. This can improve the quality of life and help individuals maintain a more consistent daily routine.

Essential Tips for Following a Low Residue Diet

Following a low residue diet can be highly beneficial for managing digestive disorders, but it requires careful planning and adherence to certain guidelines to ensure nutritional balance and effectiveness. Here are some essential tips for successfully following a low residue diet:

1. Choose Low-Fiber Grains: Opt for refined grains like white bread, white rice, and pasta made from refined flour. Avoid whole grains, which are high in fiber and can exacerbate digestive symptoms. These refined options are easier to digest and help minimize stool bulk.

2. Focus on Well-Cooked Vegetables: Select vegetables that are low in fiber and cook them thoroughly to make them easier to digest. Examples include carrots, zucchini, and peeled potatoes. Steaming, boiling, or baking vegetables until they are soft can reduce their fiber content and aid in digestion.

3. Select Tender Proteins: Incorporate lean, tender proteins such as chicken, turkey, fish, and eggs into your diet. These protein sources are low in fiber and provide essential

nutrients without adding digestive strain. Avoid fatty cuts of meat and processed meats that may be harder to digest.

4. Limit Dairy Intake: While dairy products are generally low in fiber, some individuals may find them difficult to digest. Consume dairy in moderation and choose lactose-free options if lactose intolerance is a concern. Yogurt and hard cheeses are often better tolerated than milk.

5. Avoid High-Fiber Fruits: Stick to low-fiber fruits like bananas, melons, and canned peaches or pears without skins. Avoid fruits with seeds, skins, or high fiber content such as berries, apples, and oranges. These fruits are easier on the digestive system and help maintain nutritional balance.

6. Stay Hydrated: Drinking plenty of fluids is essential when following a low residue diet. Water, clear broths, and herbal teas are good choices. Adequate hydration helps maintain digestive health and prevents constipation, which can be a concern when fiber intake is reduced.

7. Read Food Labels Carefully: Pay attention to food labels to identify hidden sources of fiber. Many processed foods and snacks contain added fiber, which can be detrimental to

your diet. Look for products specifically labeled as low fiber or low residue.

8. Introduce Changes Gradually: If you're transitioning to a low residue diet, make changes gradually to give your digestive system time to adjust. Slowly reducing high-fiber foods and incorporating low-fiber alternatives can help prevent digestive discomfort and make the transition smoother.

9. Monitor Symptoms and Adjust: Keep track of your symptoms and dietary intake to understand how different foods affect your digestion. This can help you identify specific triggers and tailor your diet accordingly. Consulting with a healthcare provider or dietitian can provide additional guidance and support.

10. Ensure Nutritional Balance: While following a low residue diet, it's important to maintain a balanced intake of essential nutrients. Consider taking supplements to cover any potential deficiencies, particularly vitamins and minerals commonly found in high-fiber foods. Professional advice can help you determine the right supplements for your needs.

Foods to Avoid and Foods to Eat on a Low Residue Diet

A low residue diet is crucial for managing certain digestive disorders by reducing the amount of undigested food passing through the intestines. Understanding which foods to avoid and which to include can significantly enhance the effectiveness of this diet.

Foods to Avoid

1. High-Fiber Grains and Cereals: Whole grains such as brown rice, whole wheat bread, bran cereals, and oatmeal are high in fiber and should be avoided. These foods increase stool bulk and can aggravate symptoms like bloating and diarrhea.
2. Raw Fruits and Vegetables: Many raw fruits and vegetables, especially those with skins, seeds, or high fiber content, can be difficult to digest. Avoid fruits like apples, berries, oranges, and vegetables like broccoli, cauliflower, and raw greens. These can cause gas, bloating, and increased stool volume.

3. Nuts and Seeds: Nuts, seeds, and foods containing them are high in fiber and can be hard to digest. This includes whole nuts, nut butters with seeds, and items like granola bars or breads containing seeds. These can irritate the intestines and increase stool bulk.

4. Legumes: Beans, lentils, and peas are rich in fiber and can cause gas and bloating. Avoid all varieties, including chickpeas, black beans, and lentil soups. These legumes are also known to exacerbate symptoms in people with digestive issues.

5. Tough Meats and Processed Foods: Tough cuts of meat and processed meats like sausages and hot dogs can be difficult to digest. They may contain additives and preservatives that irritate the digestive tract. Opt for lean and tender cuts instead.

6. High-Fat and Fried Foods: Foods high in fat, such as fried foods, fatty meats, and creamy sauces, can slow digestion and increase the risk of gastrointestinal discomfort. These foods are often harder to digest and can exacerbate symptoms like nausea and abdominal pain.

7. Whole Dairy Products: While dairy can be part of a low residue diet, whole milk and high-fat dairy products can be

problematic for some individuals. They may cause bloating and diarrhea, especially in those who are lactose intolerant. Stick to low-fat or lactose-free options.

Foods to Eat

1. Refined Grains: White bread, white rice, and refined pasta are staples of a low residue diet. These foods are low in fiber and easy to digest, helping to minimize stool volume and reduce digestive strain. Opt for enriched versions to ensure adequate nutrient intake.
2. Cooked and Peeled Vegetables: Vegetables like carrots, zucchini, and potatoes can be included if they are cooked and peeled. Cooking them until they are soft reduces their fiber content and makes them easier to digest. Avoid adding too much butter or oil, which can add unnecessary fat.
3. Tender Proteins: Lean meats like chicken, turkey, and fish, as well as eggs, are excellent sources of protein on a low residue diet. These proteins are low in fiber and easy to digest, providing essential nutrients without causing digestive discomfort.

4. Low-Fiber Fruits: Fruits like bananas, melons, and canned fruits without skins (such as peaches and pears) are suitable choices. These fruits are low in fiber and provide vitamins and minerals while being gentle on the digestive system.

5. Dairy in Moderation: Low-fat dairy products, such as yogurt, cottage cheese, and hard cheeses, can be included in moderation. If lactose intolerance is an issue, opt for lactose-free versions to avoid digestive upset.

6. Clear Broths and Soups: Clear broths and soups made from allowed ingredients (such as chicken broth or vegetable broth with cooked vegetables) are easy to digest and can provide hydration and nutrients without adding fiber.

7. Simple Snacks: Low-fiber snacks such as plain crackers, pretzels, and rice cakes can be included. These snacks are easy to digest and can be helpful for maintaining energy levels between meals.

Breakfast Delights for Low Residue Diet

Starting your day with a nutritious and delicious breakfast is important, especially when following a low residue diet. Here are some delightful breakfast options that are easy on the digestive system and perfect for maintaining your energy levels throughout the morning.

1. Smooth and Creamy Oatmeal: Oatmeal, when prepared properly, can be a gentle and soothing breakfast choice. Opt for instant or quick oats rather than steel-cut or whole oats to keep the fiber content low. Cook the oats with plenty of water or milk until they are smooth and creamy. Add a touch of honey or maple syrup for sweetness and a sprinkle of cinnamon for flavor. Avoid adding fibrous fruits or nuts; instead, a dollop of yogurt can add creaminess without increasing fiber.

2. Fluffy Scrambled Eggs: Scrambled eggs are a classic low residue breakfast option. They are easy to digest and provide a good source of protein. To make them extra

fluffy, whisk the eggs with a bit of milk or cream before cooking. Use a non-stick pan and cook the eggs over low heat, stirring gently until they reach the desired consistency. You can enhance the flavor with a pinch of salt and pepper, but avoid adding high-fiber ingredients like onions or bell peppers.

3. Banana Pancakes: Banana pancakes are a delicious way to enjoy a low residue breakfast. Use ripe bananas to make the pancakes naturally sweet and moist. Mix mashed bananas with eggs and a bit of refined flour to create a simple batter. Cook the pancakes on a non-stick skillet until golden brown. Serve with a drizzle of maple syrup or a small amount of butter. These pancakes are gentle on the digestive system and provide a satisfying start to your day.

4. Berry Smoothie Bowls: Smoothie bowls can be modified to fit a low residue diet by using low-fiber fruits and straining out any seeds. Blend a mixture of bananas, peeled and seeded apples, and a small amount of yogurt or lactose-free milk until smooth. Pour the smoothie into a bowl and top with a few slices of banana or a sprinkle of cinnamon.

Avoid high-fiber toppings like granola or seeds to keep the bowl easy to digest.

5. Rice Pudding with Cinnamon: Rice pudding is a comforting and easy-to-digest breakfast option. Use white rice and cook it in plenty of water or milk until it reaches a soft and creamy consistency. Sweeten the pudding with a bit of sugar and flavor it with a generous amount of cinnamon. This dish can be served warm or cold, making it a versatile choice for any morning. It's a satisfying way to enjoy a filling breakfast without adding extra fiber.

Lunch Favorites for a Low Residue Diet

1. Creamy Chicken Soup: Creamy chicken soup is a comforting and nourishing option for a low residue lunch. Start by cooking chicken breasts until tender, then shred the meat into bite-sized pieces. Use a low-sodium chicken broth as the base and add finely chopped, well-cooked

vegetables like carrots and peeled potatoes. To achieve a creamy consistency, incorporate a splash of heavy cream or blend some of the cooked vegetables into the broth. This soup is soothing and gentle on the stomach, providing warmth and satisfaction.

2. Tender Turkey Wraps: Tender turkey wraps are a versatile and easy-to-digest lunch choice. Use soft, white flour tortillas as the base and fill them with thinly sliced turkey breast. For added flavor, include a small amount of mayonnaise or a light dressing. You can add a slice of cheese and a few pieces of well-cooked, peeled vegetables, such as cucumber or zucchini, to enhance the texture and taste. These wraps are quick to prepare and make for a convenient, low-fiber meal.

3. Low-Residue Tuna Salad: Tuna salad can be a nutritious and filling lunch option when prepared correctly. Mix canned tuna with mayonnaise and a touch of lemon juice for added zest. Avoid adding high-fiber ingredients like celery or onions; instead, incorporate finely chopped, well-cooked carrots or peeled, seeded cucumbers. Serve the tuna

salad on a bed of iceberg lettuce or between slices of white bread. This dish is protein-rich and gentle on the digestive system.

4. Soft White Bread Sandwiches: Soft white bread sandwiches are a staple for a low residue diet. Choose soft, white bread and fill it with easily digestible ingredients like thinly sliced deli meats (turkey, chicken, or ham), cheese, and a light spread of mayonnaise or mustard. Avoid adding fibrous vegetables like lettuce or tomatoes. Instead, use a thin layer of peeled, cooked vegetables if desired. These sandwiches are simple, satisfying, and perfect for a low-fiber lunch.

5. Gentle Lentil Soup: Lentil soup can be part of a low residue diet when prepared with care. Use red or yellow lentils, as they tend to be lower in fiber and cook them thoroughly until they are very soft. Incorporate a clear broth and add well-cooked, peeled vegetables like carrots and potatoes. To make the soup gentler on the digestive system, you can blend it to a smooth consistency. This soup

is hearty and nourishing, providing a comforting meal that is easy to digest.

Dinner Ideas for a Low Residue Diet

1. Baked Lemon Chicken: Baked lemon chicken is a flavorful and tender dish that is easy on the digestive system. Start by marinating chicken breasts in a mixture of lemon juice, olive oil, and a pinch of salt and pepper. Bake the chicken in the oven until it is cooked through and juicy. The acidity of the lemon not only adds a bright flavor but also helps to tenderize the meat. Serve the chicken with a side of well-cooked, peeled vegetables such as carrots or zucchini for a complete, low-fiber meal.

2. Soft Beef Stroganoff: Beef stroganoff, when prepared with tender cuts of beef, is a comforting and hearty dinner option. Use lean cuts like sirloin or tenderloin, and cook the beef until it is very tender. Create a creamy sauce with sour cream or heavy cream, and add well-cooked, finely

chopped mushrooms for additional flavor. Serve the stroganoff over white rice or refined pasta to keep the fiber content low. This dish is rich and satisfying, making it an excellent choice for a low residue dinner.

3. Creamy Mashed Potatoes: Creamy mashed potatoes are a classic side dish that fits well within a low residue diet. Use peeled, white potatoes and cook them until they are very soft. Mash the potatoes with a generous amount of butter and a splash of milk or cream until they reach a smooth, creamy consistency. Season with a pinch of salt and pepper. These mashed potatoes are gentle on the digestive system and pair well with a variety of main dishes.

4. Steamed White Rice with Herbs: Steamed white rice is a staple of a low residue diet due to its low fiber content and easy digestibility. Cook the rice using a rice cooker or on the stovetop until it is soft and fluffy. To add flavor without adding fiber, mix in some finely chopped, fresh herbs like parsley or dill. The herbs provide a subtle, aromatic touch that enhances the rice without causing digestive discomfort.

This dish can be paired with any protein or vegetable dish for a balanced meal.

5. Gentle Baked Fish Fillets: Baked fish fillets are light, nutritious, and easy to digest. Choose mild fish like cod, haddock, or sole, and bake them with a drizzle of olive oil and a sprinkle of salt and pepper. For added flavor, you can use a squeeze of lemon juice and a few fresh herbs like dill or parsley. Serve the fish with a side of steamed white rice or creamy mashed potatoes. This dish is not only delicious but also rich in protein and healthy fats, making it an ideal choice for a low residue dinner.

Snack Options for a Low Residue Diet

1. Applesauce Cups: Applesauce cups are an excellent snack option for a low residue diet. They are made from cooked apples, which are low in fiber and easy to digest. Opt for unsweetened applesauce to avoid added sugars, and look for individual cups for convenience. Applesauce is

smooth and soothing on the stomach, making it an ideal choice for a ▢uick and gentle snack.

2. Soft Cheese and Crackers: Soft cheese and crackers provide a tasty and satisfying snack that is easy on the digestive system. Choose low-fiber crackers, such as those made from refined flour, and pair them with soft cheeses like cream cheese, brie, or mozzarella. These cheeses are low in fiber and high in protein, making them a great snack option. This combination is both nutritious and easy to digest, offering a perfect balance of flavors and textures.

3. Smooth Yogurt with Honey: Smooth yogurt with honey is a nutritious and delicious snack for a low residue diet. Opt for plain, low-fat yogurt without added fruit or seeds. Add a drizzle of honey for natural sweetness and an extra touch of flavor. Yogurt is a good source of protein and probiotics, which can aid in digestion. This snack is creamy and soothing, making it a great choice for those looking to maintain digestive comfort.

4. Rice Cakes with Peanut Butter: Rice cakes with peanut butter are a crunchy and satisfying snack that fits well within a low residue diet. Choose plain rice cakes made from white rice, and spread a thin layer of smooth peanut butter on top. Peanut butter provides protein and healthy fats, while rice cakes are low in fiber and easy to digest. This combination offers a balanced snack that is both tasty and gentle on the stomach.

5. Tender Avocado Toast: Tender avocado toast can be adapted to fit a low residue diet by using white bread and ripe avocados. Toast a slice of white bread until it is lightly golden and spread a thin layer of mashed, ripe avocado on top. Avocados are rich in healthy fats and have a smooth texture when fully ripe, making them easy to digest. For added flavor, sprinkle a small amount of salt or a dash of lemon juice. This snack is both nutritious and satisfying, providing a creamy and gentle option for a mid-day bite.

Side Dishes and Add-Ons for a Low Residue Diet

1. Creamed Spinach: Creamed spinach is a classic and comforting side dish that can be made low residue by using tender spinach leaves. Cook the spinach until it is wilted and very soft, then blend it with a creamy sauce made from butter, flour, and milk. Add a pinch of salt and a touch of nutmeg for flavor. This dish is smooth and rich, providing a delightful addition to any meal while being gentle on the digestive system.

2. Smooth Mashed Carrots: Mashed carrots are a vibrant and nutritious side dish that is easy to prepare and digest. Peel and cook the carrots until they are very soft, then mash them with a bit of butter and a splash of milk until they reach a smooth consistency. For added flavor, you can incorporate a touch of honey or a sprinkle of cinnamon. These mashed carrots are both sweet and savory, making them a versatile and satisfying side dish.

3. Baked Sweet Potato Fries: Baked sweet potato fries can be a tasty and low residue alternative to regular fries. Peel and cut the sweet potatoes into thin strips, then bake them in the oven with a drizzle of olive oil until they are tender and slightly crispy. Season with a pinch of salt or a light sprinkle of cinnamon for a sweet twist. Sweet potatoes are lower in fiber when peeled and cooked thoroughly, making them a suitable side dish for a low residue diet.

4. Gentle Green Bean Casserole: Green bean casserole can be adapted to fit a low residue diet by using well-cooked, tender green beans. Cook the green beans until they are very soft, then mix them with a creamy sauce made from mushroom soup and milk. Top the casserole with a thin layer of finely crushed crackers instead of traditional fried onions to reduce fiber content. Bake until the casserole is bubbly and the topping is golden brown. This dish is creamy and comforting, perfect for a low residue meal.

5. Steamed Zucchini: Steamed zucchini is a simple and nutritious side dish that is easy on the digestive system. Slice the zucchini into thin rounds and steam them until

they are tender but not mushy. For added flavor, you can drizzle a bit of olive oil and a sprinkle of salt or fresh herbs like dill or parsley. Steamed zucchini retains its nutrients while being soft and easy to digest, making it an ideal add-on to any low residue meal.

Desserts and Treats for a Low Residue Diet

1. Vanilla Pudding: Vanilla pudding is a classic dessert that is both creamy and gentle on the stomach. Made with milk, sugar, and vanilla extract, this dessert is smooth and easy to digest. You can prepare it from scratch or use a store-bought mix, ensuring it doesn't contain added fibers or artificial additives. Vanilla pudding provides a comforting sweetness and a velvety texture that makes it a perfect low residue treat.

2. Soft Sugar Cookies: Soft sugar cookies are a delightful and easy-to-digest treat. Made with refined flour, butter, sugar, and a touch of vanilla, these cookies are low in fiber

and gentle on the digestive system. Avoid adding any nuts or seeds to keep them low residue. Bake until they are just lightly golden and still soft in the center. These cookies are perfect for satisfying your sweet cravings without causing digestive discomfort.

3. Baked Custard: Baked custard is a smooth and creamy dessert that fits well within a low residue diet. Made with milk, eggs, sugar, and a hint of vanilla, this dessert is cooked slowly in a water bath until it sets. The result is a delicate and silky custard that is easy to digest. You can enjoy it warm or chilled, and it can be topped with a light sprinkle of cinnamon for added flavor.

4. Gentle Banana Bread: Banana bread can be adapted to suit a low residue diet by using ripe bananas and refined flour. Avoid adding nuts or whole grains to keep the fiber content low. The bananas add natural sweetness and moisture, making the bread soft and tender. This gentle banana bread is perfect for a comforting snack or dessert, providing a delicious way to enjoy the flavors of ripe bananas in an easily digestible form.

5. Smooth Ice Cream: Smooth ice cream is a delightful and refreshing treat that can be enjoyed on a low residue diet. Opt for plain flavors like vanilla or chocolate without any added chunks or mix-ins. Lactose-free versions are available for those who are lactose intolerant. The creamy texture and coolness of ice cream make it a soothing dessert that is easy on the digestive system. Enjoying a small bowl of smooth ice cream can be a perfect way to end a meal.

Drinks and Beverages for a Low Residue Diet

1. Hydrating Herbal Teas: Herbal teas are an excellent choice for hydration and relaxation on a low residue diet. Opt for gentle, non-caffeinated varieties such as chamomile, peppermint, or ginger tea. These teas are soothing and can help alleviate digestive discomfort. Brew them lightly and enjoy them warm or chilled. Herbal teas are also a great way to stay hydrated without adding any fiber to your diet.

2. Smooth Fruit Juices: Smooth fruit juices, free from pulp, are a delicious and refreshing beverage option. Choose clear juices like apple, grape, or cranberry juice, ensuring they are 100% juice without added sugars or fibers. Smooth fruit juices provide vitamins and minerals while being easy to digest. For a lighter option, dilute the juice with water to reduce the sugar content and make it even gentler on the stomach.

3. Gentle Milkshakes: Milkshakes made with low-fat milk or lactose-free alternatives are a creamy and enjoyable drink. Blend milk with a scoop of smooth ice cream or yogurt and a touch of vanilla extract for flavor. You can add a banana or a bit of cocoa powder for variety, but avoid adding fibrous ingredients like nuts or seeds. Milkshakes are soothing and provide a good source of protein and calcium, making them a perfect treat for a low residue diet.

4. Homemade Electrolyte Drinks: Homemade electrolyte drinks can help maintain hydration and balance electrolytes, especially important during illness or after

exercise. Mix water with a small amount of salt, sugar, and a splash of fruit juice, such as lemon or lime, to create a balanced drink. These homemade solutions are free from additives and fibers found in commercial sports drinks, making them suitable for a low residue diet while providing essential electrolytes and hydration.

5. Low-Residue Smoothies: Low-residue smoothies are a nutritious and versatile drink option. Use peeled, low-fiber fruits like bananas and melons, and blend them with yogurt or lactose-free milk. Avoid adding fibrous fruits like berries or seeds to keep the fiber content low. You can sweeten the smoothie with a touch of honey or maple syrup. These smoothies are rich in vitamins and minerals, providing a gentle way to enjoy a variety of flavors while adhering to a low residue diet.

Meal Plans and Shopping Lists for a Low Residue Diet

1. 7-Day Meal Plan for Beginners: A 7-day meal plan for beginners can help you navigate a low residue diet with ease. Start your day with creamy oatmeal or fluffy scrambled eggs. For lunch, opt for tender turkey wraps or low-residue tuna salad. Dinner could include baked lemon chicken or soft beef stroganoff with sides like smooth mashed carrots or steamed zucchini. Snacks might consist of applesauce cups or rice cakes with peanut butter. This structured plan ensures you enjoy a variety of meals that are gentle on the digestive system while providing necessary nutrients.

2. Customizable Shopping Lists: Creating a customizable shopping list can make your trips to the grocery store more efficient. List out your staples, such as white bread, soft cheeses, ripe bananas, and low-fiber vegetables like carrots and zucchini. Include ingredients for your favorite low residue recipes, like chicken breasts, white rice, and plain yogurt. Keeping a running list of essentials and regularly

checking your pantry will ensure you always have what you need for your meal plan, reducing the stress of last-minute shopping.

3. Tips for Meal Prep and Storage: Meal prepping and proper storage can save you time and ensure you have nutritious meals ready throughout the week. Cook larger batches of staples like rice, mashed potatoes, and soups, then portion them into individual servings. Store these in airtight containers in the refrigerator or freezer. Labeling each container with the date and contents can help you keep track of your meals and avoid waste. Prepping ingredients like peeled and cooked vegetables in advance can also streamline your meal preparation process.

4. Adapting Recipes to Your Needs: Adapting recipes to fit a low residue diet involves making a few strategic adjustments. Replace high-fiber ingredients with low-fiber alternatives, such as using peeled potatoes instead of whole grains. Cook vegetables thoroughly to make them easier to digest. When baking, use refined flour instead of whole wheat flour. Additionally, avoid adding nuts, seeds, or

high-fiber fruits to your dishes. By modifying your favorite recipes, you can continue to enjoy a variety of meals while adhering to your dietary requirements.

Welcome to Low Residue Diet……

Low residue diet Recipes

Chicken Breast in White Sauce (Low Fat)

Ingredients
- 4 chicken breasts skinless, whole or cut down the middle
- 2 tablespoons (30 g) butter
- 2¾ tablespoons (25 g) flour
- 1½ cups less 2tbsp (330 ml) semi-skimmed/light milk or half milk half vegetable stock (and omit the stock cube below)
- 4 tablespoons white wine
- 1 teaspoon Dijon mustard
- ½ vegetable stock cube crumbled
- ¼ teaspoon onion granules
- 3 tablespoons fromage blanc/fromage frais or light sour cream
- 2-3 tablespoons olive oil or use cooking spray if you've got a non-stick pan
- pepper to taste plus a little sea salt if needed and fresh herbs for garnish

Instructions

- In a large shallow pan heat 2-3 tablespoons of oil and fry the chicken breasts for 2-3 minutes on each side over a medium heat (or until golden brown). Transfer the chicken onto a plate, cover and set aside (leave the juices, if any, in the pan).
- In the same pan melt the butter over a fairly low heat, add the flour and whisk together until a thick, smooth paste forms (this is roux).
- Add the wine, stir, then add half of the milk, increase the heat and whisk until the sauce starts to thicken. Add the rest of the milk, crumbled stock cube, mustard, onion granules, pepper to taste and continue whisking until the sauce thickens and starts bubbling up. Whisk in the fromage frais, taste the sauce and adjust the seasoning as necessary.
- Place the chicken back in the pan, coat in the sauce, cover and simmer for 10-15 minutes or until the chicken is fully cooked. Add a splash of water if needed, stir and serve immediately.

Notes

• Cooking times may vary depending on the size of your chicken breasts. If you want to shorten cooking time cut the chicken breasts down the middle before frying. You can also flatten and tenderise the chicken using a meat mallet (or rolling pin) before cooking. This will also shorten cooking time.

• The sauce will thicken after a while so add a splash of water to loosen it (stir it in using a whisk). It is important to use a whisk, rather than a spoon, to make the sauce (to ensure it's smooth).

• Gluten free white sauce: You can replace the wheat flour with corn flour (use 20 g) to make this sauce gluten free.

• Substitutions: Add half the amount of milk and top up with chicken/vegetable stock.

• Seasoning: You may not need to add any salt into the sauce as the stock cube is ☐uite salty. Add plenty of pepper though.

• Best served immediately. Leftovers can be refrigerated, covered, for up to 2 days. Add a splash of water when reheating the sauce (you may have to adjust the seasoning too).

Low fodmap chili con carne

INGREDIENTS

- 400 g (14.1 oz) lean minced meat
- 1/2 red chili pepper
- 1 tsp ground paprika
- 1 tsp cumin
- 1/2 tsp oregano
- A pinch of salt
- 2 green bell peppers
- 2 stalks of spring onion (the green part)
- 400 g (1 can) canned diced tomatoes
- 160 g (5.6 oz) canned black beans
- Optional: extra ground chili to taste
- Optional: fresh cilantro

INSTRUCTIONS

- Fry the minced meat in a pan until cooked. Deseed the chili pepper and cut it into pieces. Add to the minced meat together with the ground paprika, cumin, oregano, and salt.
- Cut the bell peppers into pieces and the spring onion into rings. Add to the minced meat and bake for a few minutes.

- Rinse and drain the black beans. Add to the pan together with the diced tomatoes.
- Stir together, lower the heat, and leave to simmer for 15 minutes. Stir now and then.
- Taste the chili and season with salt, pepper and optionally some extra ground chili to taste (if you like spicy).
- Serve the chili con carne with some lactose-free crème fraîche or sour cream. I like to serve it with rice on the side, but it is also great with some plain tortilla chips or low FODMAP bread on the side. Top with some fresh cilantro.

NOTES

1. Bell pepper has been retested in 2022. Red bell pepper is low FODMAP up to 43 grams and green bell pepper is low FODMAP up to 75 grams per serving. Red bell pepper contains fructose. If you combine this with canned tomatoes in this chili recipe, your serving becomes high in fructose very quickly. If you are still in the elimination phase, I advise using green bell pepper. Green bell pepper contains the FODMAP group fructans.

Low Carb Greek Yoghurt Chicken

Prep Time: 10 minutes
Cook Time: 20 minutes
Total Time: 30 minutes

Ingredients
- Oil spray
- 5 oz. plain greek yogurt, (I used 5% fat yogurt)
- 2 tablespoon mayonnaise
- ½ cup grated parmesan cheese
- 1 teaspoon garlic powder
- 1 teaspoon salt
- ½ teaspoon black pepper
- 1.5 lb. chicken tenders (whole) or chicken breasts (cut in quarters)
- Parsley, (chopped, for garnish)

Instructions
- Preheat oven to 375°F. Lightly coat a 12 inch oven proof pan or 9×9 baking dish with nonstick oil spray and set aside.

- In a medium bowl, mix together the greek yogurt, mayonnaise, Parmesan cheese, garlic powder, salt and pepper.
- Add chicken into the bowl with yogurt mixture and coat the mixture all over the chicken.
- Move chicken to a baking dish (or oven proof pan). Chicken should be thinly coated with the yogurt mixture. Don't put too much or any additional mixture leftover.
- Bake for 25-30 minutes, or until the chicken is cooked through.
- Turn the oven to broil and place the pan under the broiler for 2-3 minutes until lightly browned on top.
- Optional: garnish with chopped parsley.

Low Carb Egg Drop Soup

Yield: 2 SERVINGS
Prep time: 2 MINUTES
Cook time: 5 MINUTES
Total time: 7 MINUTES

Ingredients

- 32 fl oz chicken broth
- 1 tbs soy sauce, or tamari
- ½ tsp ground ginger
- ½ tsp sesame oil
- 2 eggs, beaten
- 2 green onions, finely chopped
- Salt and white pepper

Instructions

1. Add the chicken broth, sesame oil, ground ginger, and soy sauce to a large saucepan. Bring to the boil, then reduce it to a low simmer.
2. Beat two eggs in a cup or bowl. Swirl the soup in one direction, and slowly pour the egg into the swirling soup.
3. Once the egg has formed into strands, add some finely chopped green onions and test for seasoning. Add salt and white pepper as necessary.

Notes

1. 4g net carbs per serving (half the recipe)
2. Only 2g net carbs if serving four people as an appetizer.

The Best Keto Cheese Sauce

Ingredients (makes about 1 cup, 4 servings)
- 1/4 cup heavy whipping cream (60 ml/ 2 fl oz)
- 2 tbsp unsalted butter (28 g/ 1 oz)
- 1/4 cup cream cheese or soft goat cheese (60 g/ 2.1 oz)
- 1/2 cup grated cheddar or hard cheese of choice (60 g/ 2.1 oz)
- Pinch of sea salt, if needed
- 2 tbsp water or more cream if you need to thin it down
- Optional: spices & herbs of choice

Instructions

1. Place the cream and butter into a small sauce pan and gently heat up. Add the grated cheddar cheese (or any hard cheese of choice) and cream cheese.
2. Stir until melted and bring to a simmer. Once you see bubbles, take off the heat.
3. Mix until smooth and creamy. If you prefer a thicker sauce, cook for 3-5 more minutes while stirring. If too thick, add a splash of water or cream.

4. Serve immediately with steamed vegetables, fish and meat. The cooled sauce can also be stored in the fridge in a sealed jar for up to 5 days.

Easy vegan chickpea curry

- Prep Time: 10 mins
- Cook Time: 10 mins
- Total Time: 20 minutes
- Yield: 4 servings
- Category: Vegan Soups & Stews
- Method: Stovetop
- Cuisine: Vegan Diet

Ingredients
- ½ red onion (chopped)
- 1 clove of garlic (minced)
- 1 tablespoon curry powder
- 1 teaspoon cumin powder
- 1 teaspoon ground coriander
- 1 teaspoon ground paprika
- 1 teaspoon dried ginger

- 1 teaspoon ground turmeric
- 1 14–ounce can of diced tomatoes
- 1 14–ounce can of low sodium or no salt added chickpeas (drained and rinsed)
- 1 ½ cups unsweetened almond milk
- 2 Tbsp maple syrup
- Salt and pepper to taste

Instructions

1. Preheat a large nonstick skillet over medium heat. While the pan is heating combine the curry powder, cumin, coriander, paprika, and ginger into a small bowl and whisk together.

2. Once the pan is ready toss in the onions and garlic along with a couple of tablespoons of water. Cook until the onions are soft. Usually, just a couple of minutes.

3. Sprinkle the dry spice mixture over the onions and garlic. Mix well until the spice mixture covers the onions and cook for one more minute. Add a little water if necessary to prevent sticking.

4. Add the tomatoes, chickpeas, and milk to the pan and stir well until everything is combined. Bring to a simmer and cook for 2-3 minutes.

5. Reduce heat to medium-low, add the maple syrup, and season to taste with salt and pepper. Simmer for 2-3 more minutes.

6. Remove from heat and serve over brown rice or enjoy by itself as a soup.

Low Calorie Chicken and Veggies Stir Fry

PREP TIME: 15 minutes
COOK TIME: 15 minutes
TOTAL TIME: 22 minutes
COURSE: Main Course
SERVINGS: 4
CALORIES: 264 kcal

INGREDIENTS
Ingredients for Stir Fry:

- 2 cups broccoli florets cut in half, see shopping tips
- 2 cups onion diced
- 1 cup carrots diced
- 5 cups cabbage shredded
- 2 cups Chinese pea pods (snow peas) sliced in half
- 1¾ cups cooked chicken breast diced
- cooking spray
- 1 tbsp vegetable, canola, or olive oil
- 3 tbsp water for stir frying

Ingredients for Sauce:
- ⅓ cup plus reduced-sodium soy sauce (for gluten free, use Tamari soy sauce)
- 2 tbsp brown sugar
- 2 tbsp rice vinegar
- 3 tbsp water
- 2 cloves garlic minced
- 2 tsp ginger (from a jar), see shopping tips
- Fresh ground black pepper to taste

INSTRUCTIONS
- First, prep all vegetables and dice the chicken. Set aside.

- In a small bowl, add all sauce ingredients and mix until well blended. Set aside.
- Coat a large nonstick wok or pan with cooking spray. Heat 1 tablespoon of oil in pan. Add broccoli, onions and carrots and water. Saute over medium-high heat for 5-7 minutes until broccoli is soft. Add cabbage and chicken. Saute another 3-4 minutes until soft. Turn down to medium heat, stir in pea pods and sauce mixture. Stir fry for about 2 minutes until all heated through. Stir constantly to blend everything.
- Store any leftovers in the fridge for a few days.

GLUTEN-FREE COCONUT CHICKEN CURRY RECIPE (LOW FODMAP + DAIRY FREE)

INGREDIENTS

FOR THE SPICE BLEND:
- 2 tbsp curry powder
- 1 tbsp paprika
- 1 tsp cinnamon
- 1/2 tsp ground ginger

- 1/2 tsp asafoetida

FOR THE CURRY:
- 1 tbsp garlic infused olive oil
- 2 chicken breasts chopped
- 200 ml canned coconut milk 180ml if low FODMAP elimination phase
- 200 ml Greek yoghurt lactose-free if low FODMAP, dairy-free coconut yoghurt if dairy-free
- 1 tbsp tomato puree
- 1 tbsp lemon juice optional
- 1-2 handfuls of spinach

TO SERVE:
- Handful of fresh chives chopped
- Fresh coriander
- Basmati rice I add 1 tsp of turmeric to mine to make it yellow

INSTRUCTIONS

- Place your pan over a medium heat and add a tbsp of garlic-infused oil. Once heated, add your chicken chunks and fry until almost sealed.
- Add your spice mix and stir fry for 1 minute.

- Next add your coconut milk and tomato puree. Stir and then simmer for about 10-15 minutes.
- Add your spinach and lemon juice, if using. Cook until the spinach has wilted down.
- Lastly, add your yoghurt and mix in.
- Sprinkle of some fresh chives and top with fresh coriander. Serve up with basmati rice and my 3-ingredient gluten-free naan bread.

Greek-Style Stuffed Tomatoes

INGREDIENTS
- 8 medium or large heirloom tomatoes or on-the-vine tomatoes
- ¼ cup pine nuts
- 1 cup chopped yellow onion
- 2 cloves garlic, minced
- 1 teaspoon dried oregano
- ¼ teaspoon sea salt
- ⅛ teaspoon freshly ground black pepper
- 1½ cups cooked short grain brown rice

- 1¼ cups coarsely chopped fresh parsley
- 2 tablespoons dried currants

INSTRUCTIONS

1. Preheat oven to 350°F. Cut a thin slice off bottoms of tomatoes so they stand upright. Slice ¼ inch off tops of tomatoes; set tops aside. Using a small spoon or melon baller, scoop out tomato pulp; chop pulp.

2. In a large, dry skillet heat pine nuts over medium 3 to 4 minutes or until golden, stirring occasionally. Remove pine nuts.

3. For stuffing, in the same skillet cook onion in ¼ cup water over medium heat 10 minutes or until translucent. Add tomato pulp, garlic, oregano, salt, and pepper. Cook 5 minutes or until garlic is softened. Stir in rice, parsley, currants, and 3 Tbsp. of the pine nuts. Cook just until rice is heated through. Cool slightly.

4. Fill tomato shells with stuffing. Place in a shallow baking dish; replace tomato tops. Spoon any extra stuffing around tomatoes. Pour enough water into dish to cover bottom. Bake, covered with foil, 30 minutes. Remove foil; bake 10 minutes more.

5. Sprinkle tomatoes with the remaining 1 Tbsp. pine nuts. Serve warm or at room temperature.

Lemon Chicken Rice Soup

Ingredients
- 1 carrot peeled, chopped
- 1 celery stalk peeled, chopped
- 1/4 cup medium grain rice such as sushi rice
- 4 cups low sodium chicken broth
- 1 cup cooked chicken breast shredded
- 3 large eggs
- 1 lemon juiced
- 2 cups baby spinach

Instructions

1. Place carrots, celery, rice and chicken broth in Instant Pot. Cook on high pressure for 10 minutes. Let naturally release 15 minutes; release remaining pressure.
2. Remove cover and set Instant Pot to saute function on high. Stir in chicken. Cook until heated through.

3. Whisk eggs with lemon juice. Gradually whisk a ladle of hot broth into eggs. Whisk eggs into soup pot. Add spinach leaves and stir. Cook until just tender

Chicken Breast in White Sauce (Low Fat)

Ingredients
- 4 chicken breasts skinless, whole or cut down the middle
- 2 tablespoons (30 g) butter
- 2¾ tablespoons (25 g) flour
- 1½ cups less 2tbsp (330 ml) semi-skimmed/light milk or half milk half vegetable stock (and omit the stock cube below)
- 4 tablespoons white wine
- 1 teaspoon Dijon mustard
- ½ vegetable stock cube crumbled
- ¼ teaspoon onion granules
- 3 tablespoons fromage blanc/fromage frais or light sour cream

- 2-3 tablespoons olive oil or use cooking spray if you've got a non-stick pan
- pepper to taste plus a little sea salt if needed and fresh herbs for garnish

Instructions
- In a large shallow pan heat 2-3 tablespoons of oil and fry the chicken breasts for 2-3 minutes on each side over a medium heat (or until golden brown). Transfer the chicken onto a plate, cover and set aside (leave the juices, if any, in the pan).
- In the same pan melt the butter over a fairly low heat, add the flour and whisk together until a thick, smooth paste forms (this is roux).
- Add the wine, stir, then add half of the milk, increase the heat and whisk until the sauce starts to thicken. Add the rest of the milk, crumbled stock cube, mustard, onion granules, pepper to taste and continue whisking until the sauce thickens and starts bubbling up. Whisk in the fromage frais, taste the sauce and adjust the seasoning as necessary.

- Place the chicken back in the pan, coat in the sauce, cover and simmer for 10-15 minutes or until the chicken is fully cooked. Add a splash of water if needed, stir and serve immediately.

Notes

- Cooking times may vary depending on the size of your chicken breasts. If you want to shorten cooking time cut the chicken breasts down the middle before frying. You can also flatten and tenderise the chicken using a meat mallet (or rolling pin) before cooking. This will also shorten cooking time.
- The sauce will thicken after a while so add a splash of water to loosen it (stir it in using a whisk). It is important to use a whisk, rather than a spoon, to make the sauce (to ensure it's smooth).
- Gluten free white sauce: You can replace the wheat flour with corn flour (use 20 g) to make this sauce gluten free.
- Substitutions: Add half the amount of milk and top up with chicken/vegetable stock.

- Seasoning: You may not need to add any salt into the sauce as the stock cube is quite salty. Add plenty of pepper though.
- Best served immediately. Leftovers can be refrigerated, covered, for up to 2 days. Add a splash of water when reheating the sauce (you may have to adjust the seasoning too).

Roasted Squash and Parmigiano Reggiano Stuffed Pasta

Ingredients
- 1 kg Crown Prince squash or other hard squash, like butternut
- 1 tbsp extra virgin olive oil
- 3 fat garlic cloves skin on
- 6 sage leaves
- 35 g dry breadcrumbs I use panko
- 100 g Parmigiano Reggiano cheese grated
- Zest of one lemon
- 8 sage leaves chopped

- 1/2 tsp nutmeg more if not freshly grated
- 175 g large pasta shells about 2/3 typical box

Marinara sauce

- 2 tsp extra virgin olive oil
- 1 small onion diced
- 2 cloves garlic minced
- 2 tbsp fresh thyme leaves or 1 tsp dried
- 700 g jarred tomatoes chopped
- 1 tsp Balsamic vinegar optional
- Salt, pepper and honey to taste

No-cook Parmigiano Reggiano Sauce

- 100 g Parmigiano Reggiano grated
- 3 tbsp créme fraîche
- 1 tbsp milk
- Extra grated Parmigiano Reggiano to serve
- Chopped parsley to serve

Instructions

- Heat the oven to 180C fan/200C/400F. Cut the s☐uash into about 8 slices, removing the seeds and rubbing the slices and garlic with the oil. Lay on a baking tray, tucking the sage leaves under. Roast in the hot oven for 40 minutes, turning once.

• Scoop the soft squash flesh into a food processor along with the garlic (pop from its skins first), Parmigiano Reggiano, fresh and roasted sage leaves, lemon zest and nutmeg. Blend just until mixed; add the bread crumbs and pulse until mixed - or hand mix them in. Scrape this mixture into a bowl and set aside. May be refrigerated and used within three days at this point.

Marinara sauce

• Heat the oil over a low-medium flame and add the onion, sauting for five minutes, stirring occasionally. Add the garlic and thyme leaves, cooking for a further two minutes. Pour in the tomatoes and their juices and cook for 20 minutes, so that it is just bubbling. Add in balsamic vinegar if using then taste for seasoning, adding salt, pepper and honey/sugar if you wish. I sometimes add a pinch of dried vegetable bouillon. Blend or mash to make it mostly smooth but with some texture. Or leave as chunky.

Pasta

• Cook pasta as directed, drain and rinse with water. Leave to cool a bit.

No-cook Parmigiana Reggiano white sauce

• Mix the ingredients together and set aside. You want a loose, pourable sauce so adjust as needed to achieve this.

Assemble and Bake

• Turn the oven down to 160C fan/180C/350F. To assemble the dish for baking, pour the marinara sauce into a shallow, wide baking dish. Take the cooked pasta shells and spoon the mixture evenly into each one, placing them in the dish as you fill them. Once filled, pour the white sauce over and bake in a oven for 20 minutes, or until the white sauce is lightly browned in patches. Pull from the oven and serve with extra grated Parmigiano Reggiano and chopped parsley

Low-Residue Turmeric Fish With Baked Sweet Potato and Avocado

Ingredients for my low-residue turmeric fish with sweet potato and avocado
- 1 sea bass fillet
- 1 sweet potato

- 1 teaspoon of dairy-free butter
- 1/2 teaspoon of turmeric
- 1/2 teaspoon of cinnamon
- 1 small piece of ginger
- 1 teaspoon of paprika
- 1 teaspoon of olive oil, or any cooking oil of choice (you could also use a low-fat cooking spray)
- 1/2 avocado
- 1/2 lemon
- Optional: 1 spoonful of sauerkraut

Directions for low-residue turmeric fish with sweet potato and avocado

1. Place fish on a baking tray and cover with 1 teaspoon of olive oil or spray with low-fat cooking spray.
2. Peel and chop avocado and place on top of fish.
3. Peel and finely chop the ginger.
4. Mix together in a small bowl: turmeric, paprika, chopped ginger, and cinnamon.
5. Once mixed, spoon over fish and ensure it's evenly coated (the oil/spray will help it stick).
6. Chop and squeeze 1/4 of lemon over the fish.

7. Cook for 20 minutes in the oven at 200 degrees.

8. The sweet potato can be baked in the oven separately – allow 40 minutes in the oven or microwave for 7 minutes.

9. One cooked, serve with a slice of lemon and (optional) sauerkraut.

10. Add the baked sweet potato as a side dish and use dairy-free butter or coconut oil for the sweet potato to soften.

Zucchini Noodles With Ginger-Peanut Sauce

Ingredients
- 3 Tbsp. natural creamy peanut butter
- 2 Tbsp. lower-sodium soy sauce
- 1 ½ tsp. freshly grated ginger
- Juice of 1 lime
- 2 tsp. pure maple syrup
- 2 Tbsp. extra-virgin olive oil, divided
- 1 (14-oz.) block extra-firm tofu, drained, patted dry, and cut into 1-in. cubes

- ½ tsp. kosher salt, divided
- 1 ½ cups matchstick carrots
- 1 red bell pepper, thinly sliced
- 4 medium zucchinis, trimmed and spiralized into thin noodles

Directions

1. In a small bowl, combine peanut butter, soy sauce, ginger, lime juice, and maple syrup, stir with a whisk. Set aside.
2. Heat 1 Tbsp. oil in a large nonstick skillet over medium. Add tofu; cook 8 to 10 minutes or until tofu is golden and crisp, stirring occasionally. Season tofu with ¼ tsp. salt; transfer to a plate.
3. Add remaining 1 Tbsp. oil to pan. Cook carrots and bell pepper until softened, about 5 to 6 minutes, stirring occasionally. Season with remaining ¼ tsp. salt.
4. Add zucchini noodles to pan; cook 2 to 3 minutes, tossing often, to heat through but not fully cook. Add tofu and half of peanut sauce to skillet; gently toss to combine.
5. Divide zucchini noodle mixture evenly between 4 plates. Drizzle remaining peanut sauce over the top.

RAW APPLE CARROT CAKE

Ingredients

1. 2 carrots, grated
2. 2 apples, grated
3. 115g pecans, finely ground
4. 85g desiccated coconut
5. 2tbsp lucuma powder
6. 2tbsp raw cacao powder
7. ½ tsp ground cinnamon
8. Pinch of salt
9. 150g raisins
10. 60g dried apple, soaked for 15 minutes
11. 60g dates, soaked for 15 minutes
12. 1 whole orange, peeled

Instructions

1. Finely grate the apple and carrots. Place in a large bowl with the nuts, lucuma, cacao, cinnamon, salt and raisins.
2. Drain the dried apple and dates and place in a blender with the orange. Process to form a paste. Add to the nut mixture and combined thoroughly. Place the mixture in

batches in a food processor and pulse to form a wet dough. Do not over mix.

3. Press the mixture into a greased, lined 20cm (8inch) cake tin and chill for 2-3 hours before serving.

RICE CONGEE

Ingredients

1. 1tbsp olive oil, coconut oil or ghee
2. 2 tablespoons minced ginger optional
3. 1-2 cloves garlic, minced -optional
4. 175g jasmine rice
5. 1600ml vegetable or chicken stock
6. 1 tsp sea salt
7. Tamari soy sauce for flavouring
8. Chopped chives for topping
9. Optional add ins – cooked shittake mushrooms, cooked plain chicken, handful of soaked sea vegetables

Directions

1. Rinse the rice with 2 changes of water. Drain and set aside.

2. Heat the oil in a large saucepan. Once hot, add the ginger and garlic and cook for 30 seconds, until they start to become fragrant. Add the drained rice, and sauté for another minute.

3. Carefully pour the broth. Sprinkle in the salt and stir. Bring the broth to a boil, uncovered. Then, turn the heat to a very low heat and cover. Let it simmer for 1 hour – do not take off the lid.

4. Turn off the heat and leave to sit for 15 minutes.

5. Serve the congee in bowls. Top with a little tamari soy sauce, chopped chives if wished.

Pasta Bake

Ingredients

1. 500 g peeled pumpkin or sweet potato cut into chunks
2. 200 g tinned asparagus cut into chunks
3. 400 g pasta
4. 50 g white bread broken up into crumbs

5. 2 tbsp oil (preferably olive oil)

6. 400 ml vegetable or chicken stock

7. 150 g grated cheese

8. 1 tsp mixed herbs

Directions

1. Preheat the oven to 220C (fan forced)

2. Place the pumpkin/sweet potato in a baking dish and drizzle with one tablespoon of olive oil and roast until the vegetables soft and golden

3. At the same time boil the pasta until al dente and drain

4. In a bowl add breadcrumbs, stock, and the rest of the olive oil, mix until breadcrumbs dissolve then add asparagus, pumpkin, mixed herbs, add pasta and mix 100 grams of the cheese through

5. Place in a baking dish and heat through for 30 minutes finish off with the last 50 grams of cheese on top of the dish for 10 minutes until melted

6. Serve with salad or steamed greens

Spinach & Mushroom Quiche

Ingredients

- 2 tablespoons extra-virgin olive oil
- 8 ounces sliced fresh mixed wild mushrooms such as cremini, shiitake, button and/or oyster mushrooms
- 1 ½ cups thinly sliced sweet onion
- 1 tablespoon thinly sliced garlic
- 5 ounces fresh baby spinach (about 8 cups), coarsely chopped
- 6 large eggs
- ¼ cup whole milk
- ¼ cup half-and-half
- 1 tablespoon Dijon mustard
- 1 tablespoon fresh thyme leaves, plus more for garnish
- ¼ teaspoon salt
- ¼ teaspoon ground pepper
- 1 ½ cups shredded Gruyère cheese

Directions

1. Preheat oven to 375 degrees F. Coat a 9-inch pie pan with cooking spray; set aside.

2. Heat oil in a large nonstick skillet over medium-high heat; swirl to coat the pan. Add mushrooms; cook, stirring occasionally, until browned and tender, about 8 minutes. Add onion and garlic; cook, stirring often, until softened and tender, about 5 minutes. Add spinach; cook, tossing constantly, until wilted, 1 to 2 minutes. Remove from heat.

3. Whisk eggs, milk, half-and-half, mustard, thyme, salt and pepper in a medium bowl. Fold in the mushroom mixture and cheese. Spoon into the prepared pie pan. Bake until set and golden brown, about 30 minutes. Let stand for 10 minutes; slice. Garnish with thyme and serve.

TURMERIC CHICKEN AND SWEET POTATO THAI CURRY

INGREDIENTS
- 2 sweet potatoes
- 2 medium sized potatoes
- 4 chicken breasts
- A handful spinach (to garnish)
- 2 tbsp olive oil

- 1/2 cup coconut milk
- 1/2 cup almond milk
- 1 tbsp chopped ginger
- 3 tbsp of thai green curry paste
- 1 tbsp of turmeric
- 1/4 tbsp of black pepper

INSTRUCTIONS

1. Peel and slice the potatoes and sweet potatoes into small chunks. Place in a pan of cold water and bring to the boil. Then leave to simmer until soft (around 25-30 minutes)

2. In a separate pan, heat olive oil and then add ginger (chopped and diced) and 3 tablespoons of thai green curry paste

3. Add coconut milk and almond milk to the pan gradually, stirring as you go to make a smooth mixture. Cook for 3 minutes to bring out flavours.

4. Dice chicken into small pieces and add to the mixture.

5. Cover chicken in the milk/curry mixture and fry on low heat for 10 minutes

6. Sprinkle over turmeric and black pepper

7. Check the chicken is cooked through (and not pink in the middle). Once cooked it should now be time to add the potato/sweet potato
8. Finally, add potato/sweet potato the pan and coat well with the mixture.
9. Take off heat and sprinkle over fresh, chopped spinach. And enjoy.

Lean Meat and Chicken Stew with Chunky Vegetables (Low-Residue Diet)

Ingredients

Lean Meat and Chicken Stew with Chunky Vegetables
1. 1 tablespoon oil
2. 4 ounces meat
3. 2 chicken thighs
4. 1 onion, diced
5. 4 cloves garlic, minced or 4 cubes Gefen Frozen Garlic
6. 1 sweet potato, peeled and chopped
7. 1 potato, peeled and chopped

8. 2 large carrots, peeled and chopped

9. 3 heaping tablespoons Tuscanini Tomato Paste

10. 8 cups chicken broth (I like to use Manischewitz Low-Sodium and add salt to my preference)

11. 1 teaspoon onion powder

12. Salt

13. Pepper

Directions

1. Heat the oil until it's screaming hot. Season the meat and chicken with salt and pepper. Add the chicken and meat to the pot and sear for two minutes on each side or until golden on the outside. Remove the chicken and meat to a plate.

2. To the same pot, add the onion, garlic, sweet potato, potato and carrots. Let them sauté until they start getting soft (do not cook them through at this point). Add tomato paste and let it cook for two more minutes. Add the chicken broth, onion powder, and salt and pepper to taste. Bring to a boil. Reduce the heat and let it simmer for two to four hours. The longer it sits, the better the flavor!

Healthy Low Fat Fried Rice

Ingredients
- Low-fat cooking spray
- 3 eggs plus 2 egg whites lightly beaten
- Ground black pepper
- 2 cups long-grain rice cooked and chilled
- 7 water chestnuts sliced
- 1 tablespoon anchovy paste
- 1 tablespoon light soy sauce or more depending on taste
- 1 tablespoon light-dark soy sauce
- 2 spring onions trimmed and sliced into rounds
- 1 cup leftover or cooked chicken or whatever meat you want to use

Instructions
- Heat a non-stick wok until hot and coat with cooking spray.
- Pour in the eggs and scramble, scraping the bits that stick to the wok. Once cooked, remove from the wok and set aside.
- Add a bit more cooking spray to the wok. Add spring onions and anchovy paste and heat through.

- Add the rice, scraping the bottom of the wok and tossing the rice until it's heated through.
- Once the rice is hot, add the remaining ingredients (including the eggs), Continue to cook over medium heat, mixing continuously for 2- 3 minutes.
- Taste and season with pepper and any additional soy sauce that may be needed.

Stir-Fry Velveted Chicken and Vegetables

Ingredients

Velveted Chicken

- 1 pound boneless skinless chicken breast
- 1/2 teaspoon salt
- 1 tablespoon rice wine
- 1 large egg white
- 1 tablespoon cornstarch
- 2 tablespoons oil

Vegetables

- 3 cups chicken broth or water

- 1 carrot peeled, cut into 1/2" thick slices
- 4 shitake mushrooms stems removed, quartered
- 1 medium zucchini peeled, seeds scooped out, sliced into 1/2" thick slices
- 1 bunch asparagus tips

Stir-Fry Sauce

- 1 tablespoon soy sauce
- 1 tablespoon oyster sauce
- 1 tablespoon rice wine
- 1/2 teaspoon sugar
- 2 teaspoons cornstarch dissolved in 2 tablespoons cold water
- 2 teaspoons sesame oil

Stir-Fry

- 2 teaspoons oil
- 1 slice ginger peeled, finely minced
- 1/4 cup low sodium chicken stock

Instructions

Velveting Chicken

1. Cut chicken into thin slices, small cubes, or thin strips. Place in bowl and add salt and rice wine; mix well. Whisk

egg white with fork until gel is broken down. Add to chicken, along with cornstarch; mix well. Add 1 tablespoons of oil and stir until well mixed. Cover and refrigerate for at least 30 minutes.

2. Bring 1 quart of water to a boil. Add 1 tablespoon oil and reduce heat to low. Transfer chicken into pot and stir to separate pieces. Continue to stir until coating turns white. Then immediately strain in colander.

Cooking Vegetables

1. Bring chicken broth to a boil in a saucepan. Add carrot slices. Cook until tender. Remove from pan with slotted spoon. Add mushrooms and zucchini to chicken broth and cook until tender. Remove from pan with slotted spoon. Add asparagus tips to pan and cook until tender. Remove from pan with slotted spoon. Reserve 1/4 chicken broth stir-fry; store remaining broth for another use

Sauce

1. In a small bowl, mix together Stir-Fry Sauce ingredients.

Stir-Frying Chicken and Vegetables

1. Heat oil in a wok or large skillet. Add ginger and stir-fry briefly until fragrant. Add cooked vegetables to wok. place

velveted chicken on top. Add 1/4 cup chicken stock to wok and cover. Cook on high for 1 minute.

2. Add Stir-Fry Sauce and toss well for 1 minute to coat chicken and vegetables with sauce. Serve

Fruity sponge cake

Ingredients
- Butter or oil, for greasing
- 50g plain flour
- 3 tbsp cornflour
- 1 tsp baking powder
- 4 eggs, separated
- 175g caster sugar

For the filling
- 295g can mandarin segment, drained
- 200g tub low-fat fromage frais
- icing sugar, for dusting

Method
- STEP 1: Heat oven to 180C/fan 160C/gas 4. Grease then line the base and sides of 2 x 20cm sandwich tins with

greaseproof paper. Sieve the flours and baking powder together.

• STEP 2: Use electric hand beaters to whisk the egg whites until stiff, then briefly whisk in the sugar. Beat the egg yolks quickly, then whisk into the whites. Fold in the dry ingredients using a large metal spoon, then spoon the mixture into the tins and level the tops. Bake for 18-20 mins until risen, light golden and a skewer inserted into the middle comes out clean. Cool in the tins for 10 mins, then gently remove and leave to cool completely.

• STEP 3: Mix the mandarins and fromage frais together. Peel away the greaseproof paper, sandwich the cakes with the mandarin mix, then dust with the icing sugar to serve. Best eaten on the day it's made.

Low Residue Low Fiber Chicken Vegetable Pasta Soup

Cook Time 30 minutes
Total Time 30 minutes
Servings 4
Calories 116 kcal

Ingredients

- 5 cups low sodium chicken broth
- 1 carrot chopped
- 1 potato chopped
- 1/2 cup tomato flesh no skin or seeds
- 1 bunch asparagus tips
- 1/2 cup cooked pastini or other small pasta

Instructions

1. Place broth, carrot and potato in a small saucepan. Bring to a boil, then reduce heat and cook until vegetables are very tender. Add tomatoes and asparagus tips and cook until asparagus is tender. Stir in cooked pasta and cook until heated through.

Greek Yogurt Fettuccini Alfredo

Yield: Serves 8
Prep time: 10 minutes
Cook time: 15 minutes

Total time: 25 minutes

Ingredients
1. 1 pound fettuccini
2. 1½ cups whole-milk Greek yogurt
3. ½ cup freshly grated Parmesan, plus more for serving
4. 3 tablespoons minced garlic
5. ¼ cup chopped fresh parsley
6. 1 teaspoon pepper

Instructions
- Boil pasta in salted water per package instructions. Reserve 1 cup cooking liquid, then drain.
- Whisk together yogurt, ½ cup Parmesan, garlic, and parsley. Slowly whisk in cooking liquid a little bit at a time. Add pepper. Pour sauce over pasta and toss to combine.
- Top with more Parmesan to taste and serve immediately. Pasta should register 145 degrees Fahrenheit or higher using an instant-thermometer placed in the middle of the dish.

Low-Residue Turmeric Fish With Baked Sweet Potato and Avocado

Ingredients for my low-residue turmeric fish with sweet potato and avocado
- 1 sea bass fillet
- 1 sweet potato
- 1 teaspoon of dairy-free butter
- 1/2 teaspoon of turmeric
- 1/2 teaspoon of cinnamon
- 1 small piece of ginger
- 1 teaspoon of paprika
- 1 teaspoon of olive oil, or any cooking oil of choice (you could also use a low-fat cooking spray)
- 1/2 avocado
- 1/2 lemon
- Optional: 1 spoonful of sauerkraut

Directions for low-residue turmeric fish with sweet potato and avocado
1. Place fish on a baking tray and cover with 1 teaspoon of olive oil or spray with low-fat cooking spray.
2. Peel and chop avocado and place on top of fish.

3. Peel and finely chop the ginger.

4. Mix together in a small bowl: turmeric, paprika, chopped ginger, and cinnamon.

5. Once mixed, spoon over fish and ensure it's evenly coated (the oil/spray will help it stick).

6. Chop and squeeze 1/4 of lemon over the fish.

7. Cook for 20 minutes in the oven at 200 degrees.

8. The sweet potato can be baked in the oven separately – allow 40 minutes in the oven or microwave for 7 minutes.

9. One cooked, serve with a slice of lemon and (optional) sauerkraut.

10. Add the baked sweet potato as a side dish and use dairy-free butter or coconut oil for the sweet potato to soften.

Tummy Friendly Creamy Pumpkin Soup

Prep time: 5 MINUTES
Cook time: 30 MINUTES
Total time: 35 MINUTES

Total time: 1 HOUR 10 MINUTES

INGREDIENTS

- 1 pumpkin
- 700 ml bone broth or chicken stock
- 3 tbsp Valsoia Soya Cream
- 1 small piece ginger
- 1 large carrot
- 1 medium sized potato
- 1 tbsp turmeric
- 1 sprinkle black pepper

INSTRUCTIONS

PREPARING INGREDIENTS

1. Peel and slice the pumpkin into small chunks. Set aside
2. Peel and slice carrot, potato and ginger.

USING A SOUP MAKER

1. In a soup maker, add the bone broth and chopped ingredients (pumpkin carrot, potato and ginger).
2. Add 1 tablespoon of turmeric and a sprinkle of black pepper.

3. Add 1 tablespoon of soya cream, stirring in.

4. If preferred, add a dash of almond milk for extra creaminess.

5. Cook in soup maker until smooth. Stir in remaining 2 tablespoons of soya cream and serve

COOKING ON THE PAN

1. Bring a pan of water to the boil and add chopped potatoes, pumpkin and carrots. Cook until slightly softened (approximately 15 minutes)

2. After 15 minutes, drain vegetables from water and pour in the bone broth. Simmer for five minutes.

3. Add chopped ginger, turmeric and black pepper to the broth mix. Simmer for a final five minutes.

4. Add 1 tablespoon of soya cream and then blend (using hand blender or regular blender)

5. Once smooth, stir in the remaining soya cream and serve.

Low FODMAP Potato Salad

PREP TIME: 25 minutes

COOK TIME: 25 minutes
TOTAL TIME: 2 hours
COURSE: Side Dish
CUISINE: American
SERVINGS: 8 people

EQUIPMENT
- Cutting board
- Knife for slicing potatoes
- Scissors for scallions/chives
- Medium stockpot
- Large bowl
- Wooden spoon
- Plastic wrap for covering / tupperware for storage

INGREDIENTS

Primary Ingredients
- 3 lbs. Yukon gold potatoes or potatoes of choice
- 4 cups filtered water with sprinkle of salt to boil potatoes
- 1 to 1 1/3 cups mayo of choice (I love Primal Kitchen or Chosen Foods!)
- 2 eggs hard boiled

- 1/2 bunch scallions snipped into wheels
- 1 sprinkle salt and pepper to taste

Optional Add-On's
- 1 to 2 stalks celery diced
- 1 bunch chives sliced thin for garnish
- 1 sprinkle paprika or celery salt
- 1 to 2 tablespoons plain yogurt for probiotics!

INSTRUCTIONS

- Wash, chop and boil the potatoes. Add to a medium stockpot and cover with filtered and salted water (just enough to completely submerge the potatoes underwater), then bring to a boil. Keep boiling until the potatoes are fork-tender (about 20 minutes).

- While potatoes are boiling, you can also boil the eggs if you haven't already.
- Strain the potatoes and let everything cool in the fridge for a few hours or overnight.
- Peel and chop the boiled eggs once potatoes have cooled.
- In a large bowl, gently combine and stir all the ingredients together.

- Garnish with paprika and/or chives.
- Have on the side with your protein and some veggies ofchoice at your next cookout, and enjoy.

Spanish-Style Shrimp Paella

Total Time: 45 min
Prep Time: 10 min
Cook Time: 35 min
Servings: 4 (1 1/4 cups each)

Ingredients
- 2 cups reduced-sodium, low-FODMAP chicken broth
- 1/2 cup white wine
- 10 saffron threads
- 1 1/2 teaspoons butter
- 1 1/2 teaspoons garlic-infused olive oil
- 1 cup uncooked medium grain rice
- 1 bay leaf
- 1/4 teaspoon crushed red pepper flakes
- 1/8 teaspoon salt

- 1/2 teaspoon smoked paprika
- 3/4 pound raw medium shrimp, deveined and peeled
- 1 cup diced unsalted tomatoes, undrained
- 3 tablespoons chopped fresh parsley
- 1/4 medium lemon, thinly sliced

Preparation

1. In a small saucepan, pre-warm the chicken broth and white wine over medium heat. Stir in the saffron.
2. In a 10-inch skillet with a heavy bottom, heat butter and oil on medium-low heat.
3. Add dry rice to the pan and coat the rice in butter and oil, stirring for 5 minutes or until it begins to brown.
4. Pour in the wine-broth mixture and add the bay leaf, red pepper flakes, salt, and paprika.
5. Cover and bring the rice to a boil over medium-high heat. Then reduce heat to low and simmer for 15 minutes without stirring.
6. Stir in the shrimp and fire-roasted tomatoes. Cover and cook on low-medium heat until shrimp are cooked through and water has evaporated, about 8 to 10 minutes.

7. Just before serving, stir in two-thirds of the fresh parsley. Serve with a squeeze of lemon and sprinkle the remaining parsley on top.

Cooking and Serving Tips

• Note that low-FODMAP broth is one without garlic or onion.
• Most shrimp on the market today has sodium phosphate added. Not only does excess sodium phosphate negatively affect the taste, but it can also result in very high sodium and phosphate levels in the shrimp. Read labels and buy shrimp that contains the least sodium per serving. Even shrimp sold at the fish counter has usually been processed with sodium phosphates, so ask to see those labels, too.
• Serve this paella with a tossed salad for a complete, healthy meal.

CLEAR SOUP RECIPE (CLEAR VEGETABLE SOUP)

Prep Time: 10 minutes

Cook Time: 50 minutes

Servings: 3

INGREDIENTS (US CUP = 240ML)
- 1 large yellow onion (avoid red onion)
- 1 cup celery stalks (you can also add more) chopped
- 2 carrots diced or cubed (can add more)
- 10 french beans (lesser if also fine)
- ½ cabbage diced
- 1 to 2 stalks celery leaves or coriander leaves
- 1½ cup mushrooms sliced (or ½ cup mixed veggies or broccoli)
- 8 florets cauliflower (optional)

Optional
- 1 tsp garlic chopped
- 1 tsp ginger chopped
- 1 tbsp oil
- 1 stalk spring onion greens or scallions
- ½ tsp crushed pepper or ground pepper

INSTRUCTIONS

Preparation (make vegetable stock)

• Add all the veggies except mushrooms & spring onions to a large pot.

• Pour water just enough to immerse them. I used 2½ cups of water.

• Cover and simmer on a low flame until the veggies wilt off completely and turn flavorless.

• Place a strainer over a large pot and strain the veggies.

• If you intend to eat the veggies then skip this step. Mash the veggies well & leave in the strainer for 20 mins. You will get about half cup soup.

How to Make Clear Soup

• Heat the same pan with oil.

• Saute ginger and garlic for a minute.

• Then add the mushrooms and saute well until they begin to smell good.

• Pour the strained clear soup to this and simmer until the mushrooms are done to your liking.

• If desired add some salt to taste. You can also serve the veggies on the side if you desire.

To make Chicken Clear Soup

• Add 250 grams bone-in chicken along with veggies & 3 cups water to the pot.

• Cook until the chicken falls off the bone.

• Remove the chicken aside and then strain the clear soup.

• Shred the chicken and set aside.

• Heat oil and saute ginger garlic until aromatic.

• Saute the shredded chicken and pour the clear soup. You can also saute mushrooms first and then add chicken.

• Let the soup come to a boil to bring out the flavors of ginger and garlic.

• Add spring onion greens and season with salt.

Low FODMAP Pasta Sauce

• Total Time: 20 minutes
• Yield: 8
• Diet: Low Lactose

INGREDIENTS

- 1 (28-ounce) can whole peeled tomatoes
- ¼ cup garlic-infused olive oil
- 1 teaspoon dried basil
- ½ teaspoon dried oregano
- ⅛ teaspoon red pepper flakes, optional
- Salt and pepper

INSTRUCTIONS

1. Place tomatoes, olive oil, basil, oregano, and optional red pepper flakes in a blender. Pulse until your desired sauce consistency is achieved.

2. Pour sauce into a large saucepan and heat over medium-high heat. Bring to a boil. Reduce heat to medium-low and simmer, stirring occasionally, for 10 minutes. Season with salt and pepper. Add more basil, oregano, or red pepper flakes, if desired.

3. Serve warm over your favorite low FODMAP pasta.

NOTES

1. Whole Peeled Tomatoes: A low FODMAP serving is a ½ cup or 92 grams. This pasta sauce makes about 8 servings, which works out to be ~99 grams of canned tomatoes. Although this is a slightly larger amount than

recommended for a green serve, it may be tolerated. If you'd like to be safe, divide this sauce into 9 or 10 servings instead.

Low Residue Low Fiber Chicken Vegetable Pasta Soup

Ingredients
- 5 cups low sodium chicken broth
- 1 carrot chopped
- 1 potato chopped
- 1/2 cup tomato flesh no skin or seeds
- 1 bunch asparagus tips
- 1/2 cup cooked pastini or other small pasta

Instructions

1. Place broth, carrot and potato in a small saucepan. Bring to a boil, then reduce heat and cook until vegetables are very tender. Add tomatoes and asparagus tips and cook

until asparagus is tender. Stir in cooked pasta and cook until heated through.

Low Residue Low Fiber Beet Carrot Soup

Prep Time 5 minutes
Cook Time 30 minutes
Total Time 30 minutes

Ingredients
- 4 cups low sodium vegetable broth
- 1 carrot sliced
- 1 can cooked beets not pickled
- Salt to taste
- Non-fat yogurt for serving if desired

Instructions

1. Place sliced carrot and vegetable broth in a small saucepan. Bring to a boil, then reduce heat and cook, covered, until carrots are very tender. Add beets and cook until heated through. Pour soup into a blender and puree

until smooth. Season to taste with salt. Serve with a spoonful of yogurt stirred in if desired.

Greek Yogurt Fettuccini Alfredo

Prep time
10 minutes
Cook Time
15 minutes
Total Time
25 minutes
Yield
Serves 8

Ingredients
1. 1 pound fettuccini
2. 1½ cups whole-milk Greek yogurt
3. ½ cup freshly grated Parmesan, plus more for serving
4. 3 tablespoons minced garlic
5. ¼ cup chopped fresh parsley
6. 1 teaspoon pepper

Instructions

• Boil pasta in salted water per package instructions. Reserve 1 cup cooking liquid, then drain.

• Whisk together yogurt, ½ cup Parmesan, garlic, and parsley. Slowly whisk in cooking liquid a little bit at a time. Add pepper. Pour sauce over pasta and toss to combine.

• Top with more Parmesan to taste and serve immediately. Pasta should register 145 degrees Fahrenheit or higher using an instant-thermometer placed in the middle of the dish.

Super Easy Low Residue Sweet Potato Hash Browns

Ingredients for my super simple Crohn's recipe: sweet potato hash browns
• 2 sweet potatoes
• 1 tbsp gluten-free flour (or the regular kind if you prefer)
• 2 eggs
• 2 tbsp olive oil

Directions for super simple sweet potato hash browns

1. First up, wash and peel sweet potatoes.
2. Use a grater to grate the sweet potatoes in a mixing bowl to create shredded sweet potato.
3. Use a kitchen roll or a cloth to squeeze the sweet potato to get rid of any extra water. This is important to stop them from being soggy or wet when frying.
4. Place your roll/cloth over the mix, press down hard, and squeeze! Keep doing this until the mix is dry and you think you've gotten rid of all the water.
5. Once that's done, break eggs into the bowl and then add a tablespoon of flour.
6. Mix and coat the sweet potatoes well with the egg and flour.
7. In your frying pan, add olive oil and heat.
8. Use your hands to squash your sweet potato into patty-like shapes.
9. Fry each patty for around 5 minutes until golden brown, then serve.

Super Simple Gnocchi and Avocado Bake (Low-Residue)

Ingredients for super simple gnocchi and avocado bake
- 250g of gnocchi (this is usually the size of store-bought gnocchi)
- 1 cup of smooth tomato passata
- 1 avocado mashed
- 1 teaspoon of paprika
- 1/2 teaspoon of turmeric
- A slice of lemon
- A handful of dairy-free grated cheese

Method for super simple gnocchi and avocado bake
1. Boil gnocchi in pan for around 3 minutes; until boiled and gnocchi rises to the top and has softened.
2. Drain the water and pour it out into an oven dish.
3. Stir in the tomato passata and coat gnocchi well.
4. Peel, slice and mash 1 avocado well and stir in with passata and gnocchi.
5. Add turmeric and paprika, coating well.
6. Sprinkle over the dairy-free grated cheese.

7. Cook for 15 minutes, until cheese melts. (The gnocchi is already cooked).

8. S◻ueeze over a slice of lemon and serve.

Healthy Fried Rice Recipe

Ingredients

- 1 tablespoon avocado oil (or other healthy cooking oil), divided
- 3 large eggs
- 5–6 scallions (aka green onions), root and 2 inches of green top removed, chopped (about 1/2 cup)
- 1 large carrot, shredded or julienned (about 1/2 cup)
- 1/2 cup frozen peas
- 2 cups cooked brown rice
- 3 tablespoons organic tamari or low sodium soy sauce
- 1 teaspoon rice vinegar (no sugar added)
- 1 teaspoon toasted sesame oil
- 1/2 teaspoon freshly grated ginger
- Big pinch of sea salt (more or less to taste)
- A few spins freshly ground black pepper

Instructions

1. Heat 1/2 tablespoon oil over medium heat.

2. In a mixing bowl, whisk the eggs into a uniform mixture until well combine and season with a small pinch of sea salt and fresh black pepper.

3. Add the eggs to the pan and scramble. Once cooked remove the scrambled eggs from the pan to a plate and reserve for later.

4. Add the remaining 1/2 tablespoon oil to the pan over medium heat; add the scallions and carrot and sauté 3-4 minutes until softened.

5. Add the frozen peas to the pan, then add the rice, tamari, rice vinegar, toasted sesame oil and ginger. Stir well to combine, the heat from the pan will quickly defrost the peas.

6. Turn off the heat and stir in the scrambled eggs. Season with a pinch of sea salt if needed–it will depend on the sodium content of the tamari and other ingredients.

7. Turn the heat to low and cook another 5 minutes until the entire dish is warmed through.

8. Water chestnuts, bean sprouts, edamame, just about any other veggie you like, or plain shredded chicken would also be a delicious addition to this dish.

Low FODMAP Cottage Pie

Ingredients for low FODMAP cottage pie
- 1 tablespoon onion infused oil
- 1 tablespoon garlic infused oil
- 1 large carrot peeled and chopped
- 1 medium zucchini, chopped
- 1 celery stalk, chopped (this small quantity of celery per serving is low FODMAP)
- ½ teaspoon dried thyme
- 2 lbs lean ground beef
- 4 tablespoons low FODMAP gravy powder (make sure the ingredients are low FODMAP)
- 1 cup beef or vegetable stock
- 1 large can chopped tomatoes

- salt and pepper to taste
- 2 cups cheddar cheese, grated

Ingredients for the mashed potato
- 1 tablespoon salt
- 2.2 pounds or about 12 medium size potatoes that are most suitable for mashing, peeled and quartered in even size
- 8 tablespoons butter, softened but not melted (or non-dairy alternative)
- 1 cup lactose free milk, warm to hot (or other low FODMAP non dairy alternatives like rice milk, almond/coconut milk etc.)

Directions for low FODMAP cottage pie
1. Heat the onion and garlic infused oils in a large non sticky pan.
2. Stir fry the chopped carrot, zucchini and celery stalk for a few minutes until softened.
3. Add the minced beef and stir with a wooden spoon to break up any lumps.
4. Cook until the meat is browned.

5. Add gravy powder and stir well.

6. Add stock liquid and stir well.

7. Add canned chopped tomato.

8. Add thyme.

9. Add salt and pepper to taste.

10. Stir well and simmer on low-medium heat for about 30 minutes or until thickened, stirring regularly.

11. Spoon meat into a large casserole dish.

12. Sprinkle half the cheese on the meat.

13. Using a pipe or just a spoon cover evenly with mashed potatoes.

14. Sprinkle the other half of the cheese on the potatoes.

15. Preheat oven to 390 F fan-forced and cook for around 30 mins, or until the mashed potato topping is of a lovely golden brown colour.

Directions for the mashed potato

1. While the meat is cooking, start the mashed potatoes.

2. Peel the potatoes and rinse them under cold water.

3. In a large saucepan, cover the potatoes with cold water, add salt in the water and bring to the boil.

4. Turn the heat down and simmer until tender (after approximately 12 minutes insert a knife in one of the potatoes to see if it's cooked all the way through).

5. Drain well and mash immediately using a masher.

6. Incorporate the butter, using a spoon and stir vigorously.

7. Slowly add the hot milk until the right consistency is reached.

8. Add salt to taste and set aside for a minute while you put the cooked meat onto a casserole dish.

Roasted asparagus

INGREDIENTS
- 500 g asparagus
- 2 tablespoon olive oil
- good pinch salt and pepper
- fresh lemon for squeezing – optional

INSTRUCTIONS
- Preheat the oven to 200°C (400°F).
- Snap the woody ends off the asparagus and discard. Wash the spears well.

- Spread the asparagus out on a large baking tray. Drizzle over the oil and season with the salt and pepper. Use your hands to toss the asparagus in the oil until they are coated, then spread out in a single layer.
- Roast the asparagus at 200°C (400°F) until cooked and just beginning to char. This will be approx. 8-10 minutes for thin spears, 10-12 minutes for thicker asparagus.
- Pile onto a serving dish, squeeze over some fresh lemon juice if you're using it, and eat hot.

Low fodmap pasta sauce

INGREDIENTS

- 1 (28-ounce) can whole peeled tomatoes
- ¼ cup garlic-infused olive oil
- 1 teaspoon dried basil
- ½ teaspoon dried oregano
- ⅛ teaspoon red pepper flakes, optional
- Salt and pepper

INSTRUCTIONS

1. Place tomatoes, olive oil, basil, oregano, and optional red pepper flakes in a blender. Pulse until your desired sauce consistency is achieved.

2. Pour sauce into a large saucepan and heat over medium-high heat. Bring to a boil. Reduce heat to medium-low and simmer, stirring occasionally, for 10 minutes. Season with salt and pepper. Add more basil, oregano, or red pepper flakes, if desired.

3. Serve warm over your favorite low FODMAP pasta.

NOTES

1. Whole Peeled Tomatoes: A low FODMAP serving is a ½ cup or 92 grams. This pasta sauce makes about 8 servings, which works out to be ~99 grams of canned tomatoes. Although this is a slightly larger amount than recommended for a green serve, it may be tolerated. If you'd like to be safe, divide this sauce into 9 or 10 servings instead.

Garlic and onion-free taco seasoning

INGREDIENTS

- 2 tablespoons ground ancho chili pepper
- 2 teaspoons ground cumin
- 2 teaspoons ground paprika
- 1 teaspoon ground oregano
- 1 teaspoon salt
- ½ teaspoon ground cayenne pepper

INSTRUCTIONS

1. Mix together ground chili pepper, cumin, paprika, oregano, salt, and cayenne pepper.

2. Store in an airtight container at room temperature until ready to use.

Low Residue Smoothie Recipes

Triple Berry Oat Smoothie

Ingredients

- 1/2 Cup(s) Quaker Oats (Quick or old fashioned, uncooked)
- 1/4 cup(s) fresh blueberries
- 1/4 cup(s) fresh blackberries
- 1/4 cup(s) fresh raspberries
- 1 small ripe banana, cut into pieces
- 1/2 cup(s) water
- 1 to 2 teaspoon(s) honey (optional)
- Cubes (optional)

Cooking Instructions

- Place oats in blender container. Blend until oats are finely ground.
- Add berries, banana and water and honey, if desired. Blend until mixture is smooth.

- For colder smoothie, add 2 to 4 ice cubes and continue blending until smooth.

Tips
- For colder, creamier smoothie, banana may be frozen before adding to blender with other ingredients.

Banana-Oat Smoothie

Ingredients
- ¼ cup old-fashioned rolled oats
- ½ cup plain low-fat yogurt
- 1 banana, cut into thirds
- ½ cup fat-free milk
- 2 teaspoons honey
- ¼ teaspoon ground cinnamon

Directions

1. Combine ingredients in a blender: In a blender, combine oats, yogurt, banana, fat-free milk, honey, and cinnamon.

2. Blend: Puree until smooth.

3. Serve: Serve immediately.

Dairy-Free Strawberry-Banana Smoothie

Total Time: 5 min

Prep Time: 5 min

Cook Time: 0 min

Servings: 2 (1 cup each)

Ingredients

- 1 to 2 cups orange juice or dairy-free milk
- 2 bananas, fresh or frozen
- 2 cups hulled strawberries, fresh or frozen
- Juice of 1 lime
- 1 tablespoon honey
- 1 tablespoon ground flaxseed (optional)

Preparation

1. In a blender, combine 1 cup juice or milk, bananas, strawberries, lime juice, honey, and flaxseed, if using.

2. Blend, adding additional orange juice or milk a little at a time, if necessary, until the smoothie is thick but pourable. Serve immediately.

Easy 5 Minute Banana Smoothie

Ingredients
- 1 banana
- 1/2 orange, peeled and ▢uartered
- 1/3 cup Greek yogurt
- 1/4 cup water or milk (dairy or non-dairy)
- 1 to 2 teaspoons honey, optional

Directions
- 1Roughly chop the banana and orange quarters, then add to a blender. Add yogurt and water (or milk).3Turn the blender on and blend until creamy and smooth.4Taste, and then adjust with honey if needed.

Banana Coconut Smoothie

Ingredients
- ¾ cup unsweetened coconut milk
- 1 small frozen banana
- 1 teaspoon honey
- 2 ice cubes
- 2 tablespoons water, as needed

Directions
1. Combine all ingredients in a blender, and blend until smooth. Taste for sweetness then serve immediately.

Banana Berry Smoothie

Prep: 5 mins
Total: 5 mins

INGREDIENTS
- 1/2 small banana, frozen
- 3/4 cup mixed berries, frozen
- 1 handful of spinach (optional)

- 1 Tbsp. almond butter or nut butter of choice
- 1/4 avocado
- 1 tsp. chia or flax seeds
- 2 scoops collagen peptides or protein of choice (use plant-based protein for vegan)
- 1/2–1 cup unsweetened almond milk or milk of choice
- 1/2 cup ice
- Optional – 1/2 cup Greek yogurt (omit for dairy-free or vegan)

INSTRUCTIONS

1. Place ingredients in a high-powered blender and blend until smooth. For a thinner smoothie add 1 cup of liquid for a thicker smoothie start with a 1/2 cup and add more until desired consistency is achieved.

Strawberry High-Protein Fruit Smoothie

Ingredients
- 3/4 cup fresh strawberries
- 1/2 cup liquid pasteurized egg whites

- 1/2 cup ice
- 1 tablespoon sugar

Preparation

1. Place strawberries in blender and blend until smooth.
2. Add all remaining ingredients and continue blending until smooth.

Banana Bread Smoothie

Ingredients
Servings: 2
Serving Size: 1 1/4 cups

- 2 medium bananas, peeled and sliced
- 1 1/2 cups ice cubes
- 3/4 cup fat-free plain Greek yogurt
- 1/4 cup fat-free milk
- 2 tablespoons rolled oats
- 2 teaspoons pure maple syrup
- 1 teaspoon vanilla extract

- 1/4 teaspoon ground cinnamon and (optional) pinch of ground cinnamon (for garnish), divided use
- 1 tablespoon finely chopped unsalted pecans or walnuts (optional)

Directions

Tip: Click on step to mark as complete.

- In a food processor or blender, process the bananas, ice cubes, yogurt, milk, oats, maple syrup, vanilla, and 1/4 teaspoon cinnamon until smooth.
- Pour into 2 glasses. Garnish with the chopped pecans and the remaining pinch of cinnamon. Serve immediately.

Healthy Chocolate Banana Smoothie

Ingredients

- 1½ cups unsweetened almond milk (or your choice of milk)
- 1 cup (packed) baby spinach
- 2 frozen ripe bananas
- 2 (heaping) tbsp unsweetened cocoa powder
- 1 tbsp chia seeds (optional, but recommended)

- ¼ tsp ground cinnamon
- 3-4 ice cubes

Instructions

1. Place all the ingredients in a high-powered blender and blend until smooth.
2. Once blended, taste and adjust according to preferences such as adding more milk for a thinner smoothie or more cocoa powder for a stronger chocolate flavour.
3. Best served immediately.

Keto Smoothie Recipe With Avocado, Chia Seeds & Cacao

INGREDIENTS

- 1–1¼ cups full-fat coconut milk
- ½ frozen avocado
- 1 tablespoon nut butter of choice
- 1 tablespoon chia seeds, soaked in 3 tablespoons of water for 10 minutes

- 2 teaspoons cacao nibs, cacao powder or cocoa powder OR 1 scoop of chocolate protein powder made from bone broth
- 1 tablespoon coconut oil
- ice (optional)
- For topping: cacao nibs and cinnamon
- ¼ cup water, if needed

INSTRUCTIONS

1. Add contents into a high-powered blender, blending until well-combined.
2. Top with cacao nibs and cinnamon.

GREEN PROTEIN POWER BREAKFAST SMOOTHIE

- Prep Time: 5 minutes
- Total Time: 5 minutes
- Yield: 2 cups
- Category: Smoothie, Breakfast, Snack, Pre/Post Workout
- Method: Blending
- Cuisine: Vegan

• Diet: Vegan

INGREDIENTS
- 1 cup (250 ml) unsweetened almond milk
- 1 ripe banana, frozen
- ½ cup (125 ml) chopped mango, frozen
- 1-2 large handfuls of baby spinach
- ¼ cup (60 ml) pumpkin seeds (pepita seeds)
- 2 tbsp (30 ml) hemp hearts (hulled hemp seeds)
- Optional: ½ scoop (approx. 30ml) vanilla protein powder and ¼ cup (60ml) water

INSTRUCTIONS
1. In a blender (or large tumbler if you're using an immersion blender) layer the spinach, banana, mango, pumpkin seeds, and hemp hearts. Add the almond milk and blend until the pumpkin seeds are really really smooth.
2. This recipe makes 1 large smoothie (2 cups - 500ml).

NOTES

1. For a nut free option, substitute the almond milk with a certified nut free oat milk, rice milk, hemp milk, soy milk, or coconut milk.

2. For a higher protein option: Add a scoop of your favourite vanilla protein powder and/or substitute the almond milk with a high protein non-dairy milk such as soy or hemp milk. This smoothie contains approx. 13g of protein when made with almond milk, substituting it with soy milk will add an additional 6g of protein. Adding protein powder will add about 6-15g of protein (depending on the brand and amount of protein powder you use.)

3. To make a variation of this smoothie without banana, substitute the banana with ⅔ cup of frozen mango or frozen peaches.

Oats Smoothie for Weight Loss

Prep Time: 10 minutes
Total Time: 10 minutes
Course: Breakfast, lunch, Snack
Servings: 1 serving

Calories: 168kcal

Equipment
- Blender

Ingredients
- 1 whole banana optional: cut into smaller chunks and frozen
- ½ cup rolled oats (or quick oats are okay if that's what you have)
- ½ cup almond milk or oat milk, unsweetened, homemade and organic, OR: Three Trees or Malk brands preferred; if you can, try to avoid all nut and oat milks with added oils and vitamins. Find the above milks in the refrigerator section of many stores.
- ½ cup water
- ⅛ teaspoon sea salt or Potassium Lite Salt

Instructions
- Add oats to blender.
- Blend or pulse until mostly powdered or finely ground.

- Add banana. (If frozen, be sure it's cut into smaller chunks or slices.) Top with milk, water and sea salt.
- Blend until smooth and creamy. Enjoy

GUT FRIENDLY SMOOTHIE

INGREDIENTS
- 1 banana
- 1 tablespoon of cashew nut butter
- 1 tablespoon of ground turmeric and sprinkle of black pepper
- 2 thumb size pieces of ginger, chopped finely and peeled
- I added these extra ingredients but these are optional depending on how you tolerate them. Although the seeds might like really tough, once they're blended in the smoothie, you should do just fine (especially with Chai since it's mainly soluble fibre. If you are cautious, then please try them one at a time.
- 1 teaspoon of Chia seeds
- 1 teaspoon of Hemp Powder

- 1/4 cup of gluten-free Muesli or oats, I used Delicious Alchemy's Gluten Free Muesli
- 1 cup of Almond Milk, I use Alpro Unsweetened because it's one of the few that are carrageenan free- but Rude Health is also a good shout

INSTRUCTIONS

1. Whizz all together in the Nutribullet for 30 seconds and voila. The perfect breakfast smoothie.

Strawberry and Banana Fruit Smoothie

Ingredients
- 3 cups strawberries, frozen, unsweetened (or other frozen fruit)
- 2 cups milk, 1%
- 1 banana, large
- 1 cup yogurt, low-fat plain

Directions

1. Wash hands with soap and water.

2. Defrost the frozen fruit just enough so that it will blend easily.

3. Pour the milk into the blender.

4. Add the pieces of frozen fruit to the milk in the blender.

5. Add the banana and yogurt.

6. Blend until smooth, about 30 to 45 seconds.

Notes

1. Strawberries, 1% milk, and low-fat vanilla yogurt used in nutrition analysis and costing.

The Best High Fiber Smoothie (Easy + Healthy)

INGREDIENTS
- 1 cup frozen mixed berries
- 3/4 cup vanilla Greek yogurt
- 1/2 banana
- 1 tbsp chia seeds
- 1/4 cup oats
- 1 cup almond milk
- 1 tsp honey optional

INSTRUCTIONS

• Add all ingredients to a blender and blend on high for 20-30 seconds.

NOTES

1. Use fresh or frozen fruit ingredients. If you use all fresh fruit, you may need a bit less liquid.
2. Course: Breakfast, lunch, Snack

Banana, oat and blueberry breakfast smoothie

Ingredients
- 1/2 cup Coles rolled oats
- 2 ripe bananas
- 1/2 cup frozen blueberries
- 2 tsp Coles Wellness Road LSA Meal (see note)
- 1 cup reduced-fat milk
- 1 cup reduced-fat plain Greek-style yoghurt
- 2 tsp honey

Method

- Blend oats, banana, blueberries, LSA, milk, yoghurt and honey together until smooth. Pour into chilled glasses. Serve.

Fruit & Yogurt Smoothie

Active Time: 10 mins
Total Time: 10 mins
Servings: 1
Yield: 1 serving

Ingredients
- 3/4 cup nonfat plain yogurt
- 1/2 cup 100% pure fruit juice
- 1 1/2 cups (6 1/2 ounces) frozen fruit, such as blueberries, raspberries, pineapple or peaches

Directions
1. Puree yogurt with juice in a blender until smooth. With the motor running, add fruit through the hole in the lid and continue to puree until smooth.

Peanut Butter and Jelly Smoothie

COOK TIME: 10 minutes
COURSE: Breakfast, Snack
SERVINGS: 1

EQUIPMENT
- Blender

INGREDIENTS
- 1 cup frozen raspberries
- 1- 1 ½ cup unsweetened nut milk (almond, hemp, cashew, etc.)
- 2-3 handfuls spinach
- 1 tablespoon peanut butter
- 1-2 dates
- 1 scoop collagen powder (I like to use Vitamin Proteins)

INSTRUCTIONS
- Add all ingredients to your blender. Start blending on a low speed and increase slowly.
- Blend until cream & enjoy.

Pumpkin and Turmeric Smoothie

Ingredients
- 1/4 cup of tinned pumpkin
- 1 banana
- 1 cup of almond milk or other dairy-free alternatives
- 1 teaspoon of nut butter (I used walnut)
- 1 teaspoon of cinnamon
- 1 teaspoon of turmeric

Pumpkin turmeric smoothie directions

This one is really simple to make:

1. Simply chop up your banana and add to your blender, along with the pumpkin, dairy-free milk, nut butter, cinnamon, and turmeric.
2. Blend until smooth.

Low Sugar Simple Green Smoothie

Prep Time: 5 minutes
Total Time: 5 minutes

Course: Breakfast
Cuisine: American
Servings: 1 -2 people

Ingredients
- 2 cups Almond Breeze Unsweetened Vanilla Almondmilk
- ¼-1/2 cup ice cubes (optional)
- ½ frozen banana and/or stevia, to taste
- 1 ½ cups baby spinach, baby kale and/or "power greens" mix
- 1 tablespoon peanut butter or almond butter
- 1 tablespoons ground flax seeds
- 1 tablespoon chia seeds
- Pinch sea salt
- Optional add-ins: spirulina or other "green" powder and/or collagen powder

Instructions
- In a blender, combine the Almond Breeze Unsweetened Vanilla Almondmilk, ice cubes (if using), banana and/or stevia, greens, nut butter, flax seeds, chia seeds and a pinch of sea salt. If using any add-ins, throw them in. Blend on

high until the smoothie is very smooth, 30 seconds - 2 minutes, depending on your blender.

• Pour the smoothie into a glass. Enjoy it right away, or let it sit for up to 1 hour before drinking (the smoothie will thicken as it sits).

Notes

Tips:

• I prefer to use baby spinach, baby kale and/or a "power greens" mix for this smoothie, which are milder in flavor than mature greens (which will overpower the other flavors).

• Almond Breeze Unsweetened Vanilla Almondmilk gives the smoothie creaminess and a delicious flavor without any added sugar.

• The ice in this recipe is optional (depending on how cold you like your beverages).

• Using frozen (instead of fresh) banana will create a richer, thicker texture, but if you don't have one you can use fresh banana instead.

• You can use either powdered stevia or liquid stevia, according to what you have and like.

- For more protein, feel free to add a neutral collagen powder.
- A green powder mix gives the smoothie a bigger boost of vitamins and minerals, but it's optional (this is the brand I use).
- A pinch of sea salt balances the flavors and provides electrolytes.

Healthy Green Smoothie

Prep Time: 10 minutes
Total Time: 10

Ingredients
- 175 g cucumber
- 45 g celery stalk
- 60 g spinach
- 100 g green apple (core removed)
- 1 kiwi fruit (skin removed)
- 150 g banana (sliced and frozen)
- 75 g pineapple (cubed and frozen)
- 3 tsp root ginger (grated)

- 2 tbsp lemon juice
- 480 ml coconut water

Instructions

- Prepare the banana and pineapple the night before and place into the freezer.
- When ready to make the smoothie, place all the ingredients into a high speed blender and blend to smooth.
- Divide the smoothie between 2 glasses and serve immediately.

Notes

1. Frozen fruit and vegetables are ideal for adding to a smoothie as they cool the smoothie mixture down, without the need for ice which only dilutes the smoothie.
2. You can replace fresh spinach with frozen spinach.
3. If there are any ingredients that you do not enjoy eating, replace them with a little extra of one of the other ingredients.

Low Sugar Simple Green Smoothie

Prep Time: 5 minutes
Total Time: 5 minutes
Course: Breakfast
Servings: 1 -2 people

Ingredients
- 2 cups Almond Breeze Unsweetened Vanilla Almondmilk
- ¼-1/2 cup ice cubes (optional)
- ½ frozen banana and/or stevia, to taste
- 1 ½ cups baby spinach, baby kale and/or "power greens" mix
- 1 tablespoon peanut butter or almond butter
- 1 tablespoons ground flax seeds
- 1 tablespoon chia seeds
- Pinch sea salt
- Optional add-ins: spirulina or other "green" powder and/or collagen powder

Instructions
- In a blender, combine the Almond Breeze Unsweetened Vanilla Almondmilk, ice cubes (if using), banana and/or

stevia, greens, nut butter, flax seeds, chia seeds and a pinch of sea salt. If using any add-ins, throw them in. Blend on high until the smoothie is very smooth, 30 seconds - 2 minutes, depending on your blender.

• Pour the smoothie into a glass. Enjoy it right away, or let it sit for up to 1 hour before drinking (the smoothie will thicken as it sits).

Notes

Tips:

• I prefer to use baby spinach, baby kale and/or a "power greens" mix for this smoothie, which are milder in flavor than mature greens (which will overpower the other flavors).

• Almond Breeze Unsweetened Vanilla Almondmilk gives the smoothie creaminess and a delicious flavor without any added sugar.

• The ice in this recipe is optional (depending on how cold you like your beverages).

• Using frozen (instead of fresh) banana will create a richer, thicker texture, but if you don't have one you can use fresh banana instead.

- You can use either powdered stevia or liquid stevia, according to what you have and like.
- For more protein, feel free to add a neutral collagen powder.
- A green powder mix gives the smoothie a bigger boost of vitamins and minerals, but it's optional (this is the brand I use).
- A pinch of sea salt balances the flavors and provides electrolytes.

Detox Smoothie

PREP TIME: 5 mins
TOTAL TIME: 5 mins
SERVINGS: 2 servings

Ingredients
- 1 cup raw coconut water or filtered water, plus more as needed
- 1 medium green apple, skin on, cored and diced

- 1 small raw red beet, peeled and diced (grated for conventional blenders)
- 1 cup frozen strawberries
- 1 cup frozen pineapple
- 1/2 small avocado, pitted and peeled
- 1 cup baby spinach
- 1 tablespoon fresh lemon juice
- Pinch cayenne pepper

Optional nutritional boosters:
- 1/4 cup frozen raw broccoli
- 1/8 teaspoon finely grated lemon zest

Method
- Make the smoothie: Throw all of the ingredients into your blender, and blast on high for 30 to 60 seconds until smooth and creamy.
- Serve: Pour into glasses and serve immediately

EASY DETOX SMOOTHIE

PREP: 5 mins
COOK: 0 mins
TOTAL: 5 mins

INGREDIENTS
- ½ cup water (or orange juice)
- 1 green apple
- ½ cup frozen pineapple chunks
- ½ frozen banana
- ½ inch fresh ginger, peeled and minced
- 1 cup fresh spinach
- Small handful fresh cilantro
- 1 tablespoon fresh lime juice

INSTRUCTIONS
- Combine all of the ingredients in a high-speed blender and blend until smooth. Pour into a glass and serve right away.
- If you don't have have a high-speed blender, I recommend blending the spinach, cilantro, and ginger with the water

first, to help break them down completely. Then add in the fruit and lime juice, and blend again.

30 Days Meal Plan for Low Residue

Week 1

Day 1

Breakfast: Smooth and creamy oatmeal with a splash of milk.
Lunch: Tender turkey wrap with soft cheese and white bread.
Dinner: Baked lemon chicken with creamy mashed potatoes.
Snack: Applesauce cup.

Day 2

Breakfast: Fluffy scrambled eggs with a slice of white toast.
Lunch: Low-residue tuna salad on white bread.
Dinner: Soft beef stroganoff with steamed white rice.
Snack: Smooth yogurt with honey.

Day 3

Breakfast: Banana pancakes with a drizzle of maple syrup.
Lunch: Creamy chicken soup with a soft roll.
Dinner: Gentle baked fish fillets with smooth mashed carrots.
Snack: Soft sugar cookies.

Day 4

Breakfast: Berry smoothie bowl with yogurt and peeled banana.
Lunch: Tender turkey wrap with peeled cucumber slices.
Dinner: Steamed zucchini with rice and tender chicken strips.
Snack: Rice cakes with peanut butter.

Day 5

Breakfast: Smooth oatmeal with a touch of cinnamon.
Lunch: Soft white bread sandwich with ham and cheese.

Dinner: Gentle green bean casserole with baked sweet potato fries.

Snack: Vanilla pudding.

Day 6

Breakfast: Fluffy scrambled eggs with a side of smooth yogurt.

Lunch: Creamy chicken soup with soft white bread.

Dinner: Baked lemon chicken with smooth mashed carrots.

Snack: Soft sugar cookies.

Day 7

Breakfast: Banana pancakes with honey.

Lunch: Low-residue tuna salad on white bread.

Dinner: Soft beef stroganoff with steamed zucchini.

Snack: Applesauce cup.

Week 2

Day 8

Breakfast: Smooth and creamy oatmeal.
Lunch: Tender turkey wrap with peeled and cooked carrots.
Dinner: Baked lemon chicken with creamy mashed potatoes.
Snack: Smooth yogurt with honey.

Day 9

Breakfast: Fluffy scrambled eggs with white toast.
Lunch: Soft white bread sandwich with turkey and cheese.
Dinner: Gentle baked fish fillets with steamed white rice.
Snack: Rice cakes with peanut butter.

Day 10

Breakfast: Banana pancakes with a touch of honey.
Lunch: Creamy chicken soup with a soft roll.
Dinner: Soft beef stroganoff with smooth mashed carrots.

Snack: Vanilla pudding.

Day 11

Breakfast: Berry smoothie bowl with peeled banana.
Lunch: Low-residue tuna salad on white bread.
Dinner: Baked lemon chicken with steamed zucchini.
Snack: Soft sugar cookies.

Day 12

Breakfast: Smooth oatmeal with a splash of milk.
Lunch: Tender turkey wrap with peeled cucumber slices.
Dinner: Gentle green bean casserole with baked sweet potato fries.
Snack: Applesauce cup.

Day 13

Breakfast: Fluffy scrambled eggs with smooth yogurt.
Lunch: Soft white bread sandwich with ham and cheese.

Dinner: Baked lemon chicken with creamy mashed potatoes.

Snack: Smooth yogurt with honey.

Day 14

Breakfast: Banana pancakes with maple syrup.

Lunch: Creamy chicken soup with a soft roll.

Dinner: Soft beef stroganoff with steamed white rice.

Snack: Soft sugar cookies.

Week 3

Day 15

Breakfast: Smooth and creamy oatmeal.

Lunch: Tender turkey wrap with soft cheese.

Dinner: Baked lemon chicken with smooth mashed carrots.

Snack: Vanilla pudding.

Day 16

Breakfast: Fluffy scrambled eggs with a slice of white toast.
Lunch: Low-residue tuna salad on white bread.
Dinner: Gentle baked fish fillets with steamed zucchini.
Snack: Rice cakes with peanut butter.

Day 17

Breakfast: Berry smoothie bowl with yogurt and peeled banana.
Lunch: Soft white bread sandwich with turkey and cheese.
Dinner: Soft beef stroganoff with creamy mashed potatoes.
Snack: Applesauce cup.

Day 18

Breakfast: Banana pancakes with a touch of honey.
Lunch: Creamy chicken soup with a soft roll.
Dinner: Baked lemon chicken with steamed white rice.
Snack: Smooth yogurt with honey.

Day 19

Breakfast: Smooth oatmeal with cinnamon.
Lunch: Tender turkey wrap with peeled cucumber slices.
Dinner: Gentle green bean casserole with baked sweet potato fries.
Snack: Soft sugar cookies.

Day 20

Breakfast: Fluffy scrambled eggs with smooth yogurt.
Lunch: Soft white bread sandwich with ham and cheese.
Dinner: Soft beef stroganoff with smooth mashed carrots.
Snack: Vanilla pudding.

Day 21

Breakfast: Banana pancakes with maple syrup.
Lunch: Low-residue tuna salad on white bread.
Dinner: Baked lemon chicken with steamed zucchini.
Snack: Rice cakes with peanut butter.
Week 4

Day 22

Breakfast: Smooth and creamy oatmeal.
Lunch: Tender turkey wrap with peeled and cooked carrots.
Dinner: Gentle baked fish fillets with steamed white rice.
Snack: Smooth yogurt with honey.

Day 23

Breakfast: Fluffy scrambled eggs with white toast.
Lunch: Soft white bread sandwich with turkey and cheese.
Dinner: Baked lemon chicken with creamy mashed potatoes.
Snack: Soft sugar cookies.

Day 24

Breakfast: Berry smoothie bowl with peeled banana.
Lunch: Creamy chicken soup with a soft roll.
Dinner: Soft beef stroganoff with steamed zucchini.
Snack: Applesauce cup.

Day 25

Breakfast: Banana pancakes with honey.
Lunch: Low-residue tuna salad on white bread.
Dinner: Baked lemon chicken with smooth mashed carrots.
Snack: Vanilla pudding.

Day 26

Breakfast: Smooth oatmeal with a splash of milk.
Lunch: Tender turkey wrap with peeled cucumber slices.
Dinner: Gentle green bean casserole with baked sweet potato fries.
Snack: Smooth yogurt with honey.

Day 27

Breakfast: Fluffy scrambled eggs with smooth yogurt.
Lunch: Soft white bread sandwich with ham and cheese.
Dinner: Soft beef stroganoff with creamy mashed potatoes.
Snack: Rice cakes with peanut butter.

Day 28

Breakfast: Banana pancakes with maple syrup.
Lunch: Creamy chicken soup with a soft roll.
Dinner: Baked lemon chicken with steamed white rice.
Snack: Soft sugar cookies.

Day 29

Breakfast: Smooth and creamy oatmeal.
Lunch: Tender turkey wrap with soft cheese.
Dinner: Gentle baked fish fillets with steamed zucchini.
Snack: Applesauce cup.

Day 30

Breakfast: Fluffy scrambled eggs with a slice of white toast.
Lunch: Low-residue tuna salad on white bread.
Dinner: Soft beef stroganoff with smooth mashed carrots.
Snack: Vanilla pudding.

CONCLUSION

A low residue diet is a specialized eating plan designed to reduce the amount of indigestible material passing through the digestive tract. It is particularly beneficial for individuals with digestive disorders such as Crohn's disease, ulcerative colitis, diverticulitis, or those recovering from gastrointestinal surgery. By limiting high-fiber foods, this diet aims to minimize bowel movements, decrease stool volume, and alleviate symptoms like abdominal pain and diarrhea. A low residue diet can be an effective tool for managing certain digestive disorders and promoting gut health. With the right approach, it is possible to enjoy a wide range of tasty and gentle foods while supporting digestive comfort and overall well-being.

www.ingramcontent.com/pod-product-compliance
Lightning Source LLC
Chambersburg PA
CBHW071830210526
45479CB00001B/77